RESEARCH AND PERSPECTIVES IN LONGEVITY

Springer

Berlin
Heidelberg
New York
Barcelona
Hong Kong
London
Milan
Paris
Singapore
Tokyo

J.-M. Robine   T.B.L. Kirkwood   M. Allard (Eds.)

Sex and Longevity: Sexuality, Gender, Reproduction, Parenthood

With 36 Figures and 21 Tables

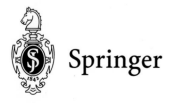

Springer

JEAN-MARIE ROBINE
Equipe INSERM Démographie et Santé
Val d'Aurelle
Parc Euromédecine
34298 Montpellier cedex 5
France

THOMAS B.L. KIRKWOOD
Department of Gerontology
University of Newcastle
Wolfson Research Centre
Newcastle General Hospital
Newcastle upon Tyne, NE4 6BE
UK

MICHEL ALLARD
Fondation IPSEN
24, rue Erlanger
75781 Paris Cedex 16
France

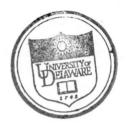

QP 85 .S38 2001 (library stamp handwriting)

ISBN 3-540-67740-2   Springer-Verlag Berlin Heidelberg New York

Library of Congress Cataloging-in-Publication Data

Sex and longevity : sexuality, gender, reproduction, parenthood / J.-M. Robine, T.B.L. Kirkwood, M. Allard (eds.). (Research and Perspectives in Longevity)
p. cm.
Includes bibliographical references and index.
ISBN 3540677402 (alk. paper)
1. Longevity-Sex differences. 2. Longevity-Genetic aspects. 3. Mothers-Mortality. I. Robine, Jean-Marie. II. Kirkwood, T.B.L. III. Allard, M., 1946–
QP85 .S38 2000
612.6'8–dc21   00-055697

Springer Verlag Berlin Heidelberg New York
a member of BertelsmannSpringer Science + Business Media GmbH

© Springer-Verlag Berlin Heidelberg 2001
Printed in Germany

The use of general descriptive names, registered names, trademarks, etc., in this publication does not imply, even in the absence of a specific statement, that such names are exempt from the relevant protective laws and regulations and therefore free for general use.

Product Liability: The publishers cannot guarantee the accuracy of any information about dosage and application contained in this book. In every individual case the user must check such information by consulting the relevant literature.

Herstellung: PROEDIT GmbH, 69126 Heidelberg, Germany
Cover design: design & production, 69121 Heidelberg, Germany
Typesetting: Mitterweger & Partner GmbH, Plankstadt
Printed on acid-free paper   SPIN: 10717976   27/3136wg – 5 4 3 2 1 0 –

Preface

In most human societies, females live longer than males, though we do not understand why this is so. Another puzzle is why some people live in good health to great ages while others die relatively young. It is becoming increasingly urgent to find answers to these questions because improved diet, public health and medicine mean that many more people will live longer, leading to an ageing of the human population. An international group of experts, hosted by the Fondation IPSEN, met in Paris in October 1999 to discuss the latest advances towards understanding why some of us age faster than others, during the third meeting of the series "Colloques Médecine et Recherche", which is devoted to "Research and Perspectives in Longevity".

The studies that follow the lives of defined groups of people over many years are important sources of information on longevity. In the Netherlands, sex differentials in survival at ages 1, 15, 40 and 50 were examined through two longitudinal studies. Both studies suggest that women have a higher chance of survival at each age, which may in part account for more women than men surviving into old age (D.J.H. Deeg, Amsterdam, The Netherlands). Another source of reliable data is the records of aristocratic families (T. Kirkwood, Newcastle upon Tyne, UK; L. Gravrilov and N Gravrilova., Chicago, USA) in which a higher fertility, i.e., more children, seems to be related to a shorter life, indicating that the available resources are distributed between the maintenance of one's own body and reproduction (T. Kirkwood).

The tendency to live longer seems to run in families. Evidence that this longevity is, at least in part, inherited comes from the study of four American families that are remarkable for their number of survivors into very old age. For example, in one family, 5 of 16 siblings became centenarians, which is highly unlikely to be a chance event (T. Perls, Boston, USA). Examination of the population register for the Valserine Valley in the French Jura in the 18th and 19th centuries has shown the sex dependence of human longevity and of its inheritance: the pattern indicates that survival beyond reproductive age is linked to the sex-determining X chromosome (A. Cournil, Lyon, France). Support for this conclusion comes from a study of European royal and aristocratic families showing that daughters born to fathers over the age of 45 were more likely to die young than were sons, implicating an accumulation of deleterious mutations on the X chromosome during the parent's life (L. Gavrilov and N. Gravrilova, Chicago, USA).

Parenthood also influences survival. It makes sense in evolutionary terms that parents should survive until their offspring is independent. A comparison of parenting and survival across several species of apes and monkeys revealed that the sex that invests most in raising the offspring lives longer. The clearest example is the comparison between the New World spider monkey, where the females do most of the parenting and live much longer, and the owl and titi monkeys, where the males do most of the childcare and considerably outlive the females (J. Allman, Pasadena, USA). In humans the pattern is less striking, perhaps because males take part of the responsibility for raising children. Child-bearing itself affects longevity in human females: women having two to five children later in their reproductive span are likely to live longer (E. Lund, Tromso, Norway). However, mothers over the age of 35 do not seem to transmit their longevity to their offspring, whereas younger mothers do (L. Gavrilov and N. Gravrilova, Chicago, USA).

Why females should survive well after they lose fertility, a phenomenon that is not unique to humans but widespread among mammals, is hotly debated. It may be an advantage to have older females in the population with time and experience to invest in the care of their children's offspring. This "grandmother" effect has been demonstrated in demographic data from the Gambia (R. Mace, London, UK).

But menopause may have had other evolutionary roots, onto which grandmothering has been grafted as a cultural development. Studies of lions and baboons indicate that the primary advantage may be to ensure that the mother survives until the last of her offspring becomes independent; the relatively early occurrence of menopause in humans may reflect the long period of infancy (C. Packer, St Paul, USA). Menopause thus seems likely to have positive functions, rather than being merely a byproduct of modern women living to greater ages. Such perspectives need to be considered seriously as techniques that artificially extend the human reproductive span are being developed. The controversial topic of countering the effects of ageing by supplementing the waning sex hormones in men as well as women is also discussed (J. Morley, St Louis, USA).

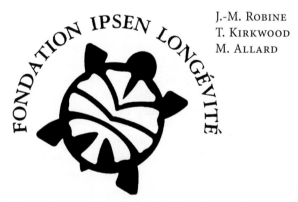

J.-M. ROBINE
T. KIRKWOOD
M. ALLARD

Acknowledgements: The editors wish to thank Mary Lynn Gage and Isabelle Romieu for editorial assistance and Jacqueline Mervaillie for the organization of the meeting in Paris.

Contents

List of Contributors

Allman, J.
Division of Biology, California Institute of Technology, Pasadena, California 91125, USA

Brewster, S.
Beth Israel Deaconess Medical Center, Gerontology Division, Rabb 417, 330 Brookline Ave, Boston, MA 02215, USA

Cournil, A.
Laboratoire "Biométrie et Biologie évolutive", UMR CNRS 5558, Université C. Bernard, Lyon 1, 43 boulevard du 11 novembre 1918, 69622 Villeurbanne cedex, France

Daly, M.
Beth Israel Deaconess Medical Center, Gerontology Division, Rabb 417, 330 Broolline Ave, Boston, MA 02215, USA

Deeg, D.J.H.
Department of Psychiatry, Institute for Research in Extramural Medicine, Vrije Universiteit, Faculty SCW/LASA, De Boelelaan 1081c, 1081 HV Amsterdam, The Netherlands

Fretts, R.
Beth Israel Deaconess Medical Center, Gerontology Division, Rabb 417, 330 Brookline Ave, Boston, MA 02215, USA

Gavrilov, L.A.
Center on Aging, NORC/University of Chicago, 1155 East 60th Street, Chicago, IL 60637, USA

Gavrilova, N.S.
Center on Aging, NORC/University of Chicago, 1155 East 60th Street, Chicago, IL 60637, USA

Hasenstaub, A.
Division of Biology, California Institute of Technology, Pasadena,
California 91125, USA

Kirkwood, T.B.L.
Department of Gerontology, University of Newcastle, Wolfson Research Centre,
Newcastle General Hospital, Newcastle upon Tyne NE4 6BE, UK

Kumle, M.
Institute of Community Medicine, University of Tromsø, 9037 Tromsø, Norway

Kunkel, L.
Beth Israel Deaconess Medical Center, Gerontology Division, Rabb 417,
330 Brooline Ave, Boston, MA 02215, USA

Lund, W.
Institute of Community Medicine, University of Tromsø, 9037 Tromsø, Norway

Mace, R.
Department of Anthropology, University College London, Gower St.,
London WC1E 6BT, UK

Morley, J.E.
Geriatric Research, Education and Clinical Center, St. Louis VAMC, St. Louis,
MO 63125
and
Division of Geriatric Medicine, Saint Louis University Medical School, St. Louis,
MO, USA

Packer, C.
Department of Ecology, Evolution and Behaviour, University of Minnesota,
1987 Upper Buford Circle, St. Paul, MN 55108, USA

Perls, T.
Beth Israel Deaconess Medical Center, Gerontology Division, Rabb 417,
330 Brookline Ave, Boston, MA 02215, USA

Puca, A.
Beth Israel Deaconess Medical Center, Gerontology Division, Rabb 417,
330 Brookline Ave, Boston, MA 02215, USA

Westendorp, R.G.J.
Departments of Gerontology and Geriatrics, and Clinical Epidemiology,
Leiden University Medical Centre C1-R, P.O. Box 9600, 2300 RC Leiden,
The Netherlands

Human Longevity at the Cost of Reproductive Success: Trade-Offs in the Life History

T. B. L. Kirkwood and R.G.J Westendorp

Introduction

A central concept in the evolutionary theory of senescence is the idea that ageing results from life-history trade-offs (Williams 1957; Kirkwood 1981; Kirkwood and Rose 1991; Rose 1991, Partridge and Barton 1993). In particular, the disposable soma theory (Kirkwood 1977, 1981; Kirkwood and Holliday 1979) suggests that longevity is determined through the setting of longevity assurance mechanisms so as to provide an optimal compromise between investments in somatic maintenance (including stress resistance) and in reproduction. A corollary is that species with low extrinsic mortality are predicted to invest relatively more effort in maintenance, resulting in slower intrinsic ageing, than species with high extrinsic mortality. Comparative studies among mammalian species confirm that cells from long-lived species appear to have a greater intrinsic capacity to withstand stresses than cells from short-lived species (Kapahi et al. 1999). Ecological comparisons support the idea that short-lived species invest in higher rates of reproduction – necessary because such species are generally subject to higher extrinsic mortality – leaving fewer resources available for somatic maintenance and repair.

It is also predicted that, *within* a species, there is likely to be an inverse correlation between fertility and longevity, provided that there is some heterogeneity with respect to genetic determinants of longevity. The existence of intraspecific heterogeneity with respect to genetic determinants of longevity is supported by data from human populations indicating significant heritability of life span (McGue et al. 1993; Vaupel et al. 1998). In the fruit fly *Drosophila melanogaster*, selection on late egg-laying capacity in females resulted in populations with extended life spans but decreased early fecundity (for reviews see Rose 1991; Partridge and Barton 1993), providing direct support for the concept of trade-offs. Furthermore, an experiment selecting directly for increased life span revealed a similar result: the long-lived populations resulting from selection for increased life span showed reduced early fecundity (Zwaan et al. 1995).

Theoretical studies of life history optimisation have shown that, although in a given environment there is likely to be a unique optimal compromise between investments in somatic maintenance and in reproduction, the nature of the optimising process is such that, within the vicinity of the optimum, the fitness peak is quite flat (Kirkwood and Holliday 1986; Kirkwood and Rose 1991). It is there-

Robine et al. (Eds.)
Sex and Longevity: Sexuality, Gender,
Reproduction, Parenthood
© Springer-Verlag Berlin Heidelberg 2000

Table 1. Variation and covariation about the optimal life history according to a model based on the disposable soma theory (Kirkwood and Rose 1991) and fitted using data for the mouse *Mus musculus*

Intrinsic rate of natural increase	Fraction of metabolic resources allocated to somatic maintenance	Life span (99th centile), months	Peak reproductive rate, offspring per month
$r = -0.001$	0.455	31	4.4
$r = 0.0$	0.5	36	4.0
$r = -0.001$	0.56	45	3.5

At the optimum, the intrinsic rate of natural increase in the population $r = 0.0$ (i.e., constant population size) and the fraction of metabolic resources allocated to maintenance is 0.5. This results in a life span of 36 months and a peak reproductive rate of four offspring per month. The table also shows the predicted life spans and peak reproductive rates for a range either side of the optimum such that intrinsic rate of natural increase decreases by a small amount (0.001). It may be seen that this range encompasses significant variation in life span and reproductive rate, with negative covariation between these traits.

fore possible to deviate from the optimum without incurring a major loss in fitness (Table 1). This tendency will be reinforced when the environment includes unpredictable variations, so that a range of optimal strategies may be found. Such variation within the population is predicted to be associated with negative covariance of fecundity and longevity.

Since the evolutionary arguments summarised above are quite general, it is predicted that these effects might also be seen in human populations. We recently carried out an analysis of human records that appear to reveal such a trade-off.

The British Aristocrats Study

There are many ways in which non-genetic heterogeneity within populations might generate positive associations between longevity and fertility. The most obvious is through variance in socioeconomic factors, particularly wealth. Poverty typically confers increased risk of malnutrition and general ill health, resulting in reduced life expectancy and a possibly greater risk of infertility. We therefore sought a population whose life history variables might be affected as little as possible by socioeconomic heterogeneity. We used records for the British aristocracy, the advantages of which are the relative completeness of records extending over a long period of history, and the unusually privileged socioeconomic status of the individuals. The latter is apparent from the fact that life span among British aristocrats began to increase (see Table 2) about 150 years earlier than in the general population of Great Britain, i.e., 1700 versus 1850 (Hollingworth 1965; Cairns 1997). A further practical advantage was that these data were conveniently available on a CD-ROM (see Westendorp and Kirkwood 1998 for details).

A striking aspect of the data was the relatively low overall fertility for British aristocrats, a feature also reported by earlier authors (see Cummins 1999). Although the low average fertility in the records for British aristocrats indicates

Table 2. Trends in longevity and fertility of female aristocrats (abbreviated from Westendorp and Kirkwood 1998)

Birth cohort	Number	Mean age at death	Mean no. of children
< 1500	337	46.1	2.34
1501–1550	106	42.9	2.31
1551–1600	122	44.7	2.03
1601–1650	190	45.8	2.83
1651–1700	296	43.1	2.41
1701–1725	124	43.3	2.22
1726–1750	120	52.3	2.50
1751–1775	149	53.1	2.19
1776–1800	174	55.3	2.20
1801–1825	222	60.5	1.76
1826–1850	216	61.4	2.06
1851–1875	385	68.0	1.54

that this population was somewhat atypical, there is no obvious reason why this should distort any trade-off between fertility and longevity.

After excluding a small proportion (< 1 %) of records because of obvious errors, we examined records for 33,497 individuals (19,380 males; 13,667 females) representing 18,125 marriages, whose dates of birth ranged from the 8th century until the late 19th century. We chose a cut-off after the 1875 birth cohort to exclude individuals who might still be living.

The relationships between female longevity (expressed as age at death in 10-year groups), proportion childless, number of progeny, and age at first childbirth are summarised in Table 3, where the data are adjusted for trends over calendar time (see Westendorp and Kirkwood 1998 for details).

Women who died young had little opportunity to reproduce and therefore it is not surprising that these women showed a high proportion who died childless, a low average age at first childbirth, and a low number of progeny. For women who died between age 31 and 60, there was an approximately constant proportion

Table 3. Female reproduction and age at death adjusted for trends over calendar time (abbreviated from Westendorp and Kirkwood 1998)

Age at death	Number	Percent childless	Mean age at first childbirth	Mean no. of children
< 20	42	66	19.1	0.45
21–30	176	39	20.5	1.35
31–40	218	26	23.2	2.05
41–50	210	31	23.9	2.01
51–60	299	28	24.6	2.40
61–70	337	33	23.8	2.36
71–80	322	31	24.6	2.64
81–90	247	45	25.1	2.08
> 90	57	49	27.0	1.80

who remained childless and an approximately constant age at first childbirth. The number of progeny showed an increase with age at death, consistent with the fact that the longer a woman lived, the greater opportunity she would have had to have children. Opportunity for having further children would have ceased with menopause.

Therefore, in the absence of any trade-off between longevity and fertility, it would be predicted that number of progeny should reach a plateau. However, the women who died at the oldest ages showed significantly reduced numbers of children, compared with those who died at earlier ages. Also, those women who died at the oldest ages had their first children at significantly later ages, consistent with the idea that they may have had impaired fertility.

While cause and effect cannot be established unambiguously from these kinds of historical data, the results are compatible with the prediction that individuals with increased predisposition to longevity have decreased predisposition to fertility, and vice versa. An alternative is that "wear and tear" associated with childbirth might explain this inverse association. Since wear and tear would affect males less than females, whereas an intrinsic trade-off between fertility and longevity would be predicted to affect both sexes, we also examined the data in a similar way for males. The results (not shown here; see Westendorp and Kirkwood 1998) showed that the apparent trade-off between longevity and fertility was strikingly similar for males and females.

The fact that similar trade-offs were seen for males and females suggested that reproductive "wear-and-tear" was not the explanation. Environmental factors could, in principle, be important, for example if a large family increased stress and mortality risk for both parents. We tested this by entering spouse's age at death as an explanatory variable that might capture any effect of environment. We found that, although the correlation between spouses was statistically significant, it explained only 2 % of the variance in age at death (Westendorp and Kirkwood 1999a), and the trade-off was unaffected. We concluded that the most likely explanation was, therefore, an intrinsic trade-off between genetic factors promoting fertility and longevity.

Subsequently, Gavrilov and Gavrilova (1999) raised a number of points about our analysis. In particular they asked whether extraneous factors might have distorted the trade-off we described or whether incompleteness in the data might have caused distortion. Gavrilov and Gavrilova suggested that, in addition to the variables already taken into account in our analysis, variation in age at marriage and spousal age difference might have distorted the relationship between number of progeny and longevity.

In a laboratory experiment, one minimizes artifact by design. With historical human data, this method of eliminating distorting variables is not available. The experimental situation can be mimicked, however, by applying appropriate exclusion criteria (Miettinen 1985, p. 57). Table 4 shows results from survival analyses (Westendorp and Kirkwood 1999b) in which we estimated mortality risk after age 60 years in married women who had had two or more children, compared to women with zero or one child. When all of the women aged 60 years and older

Table 4. Mortality risk after age 60 years in married aristocratic women born before 1876 (from Westendorp and Kirkwood 1999b)

Exclusion criterion	No.	Mortality risk (95 % CI)[a]	p-value
None	1004	1.16 (1.02–1.32)	0.02
+ Born before 1500	915	1.20 (1.05–1.37)	0.008
+ Married after age 30 years	761	1.19 (1.03–1.38)	0.02
+ Spouse aged over 35 years	505	1.19 (0.99–1.42)	0.06

[a] Mortality estimates for women with two or more children compared to women with zero or one child are adjusted over time using Cox regression; figures in parentheses denote 95 % confidence intervals.

from our original publication were analyzed, those who had two or more children had 16 % higher mortality (mortality risk 1.16) than women with zero or one child. This amounts to a mean difference in survival of three to four years. The excess mortality remained similar when the data set was progressively restricted to aristocratic women born after 1500 (to exclude the period of greatest incompleteness), then also to women married before age 30 years (to exclude the possible effect of age at marriage), then also to women whose husbands at marriage were aged less than 35 years (to exclude the possible effect of spousal age difference). Although the confidence intervals inevitably became wider as more of the observations were excluded, the point estimates for excess mortality remained remarkably constant.

Discussion

Given that there appears to be genetic variation in human populations with respect to determinants of longevity, and that there is evidence from other species of trade-offs between longevity and fertility, it seems reasonable to hypothesise that the pattern detected in the British aristocrats might reflect a general feature of human life history. However, testing this will not be easy. Variations in socioeconomic status may generate *positive* associations between life history traits. Futhermore, the actions of intrinsic chance in generating phenotypic variations that have nothing to do with genes or external environment (see Finch and Kirkwood 2000) may work in a similar direction to produce positive associations between fertility and longevity. Even with the same genotype and environment there is considerable scope for intrinsic stochastic variations affecting cell and molecular processes to produce individual variations in how the phenotype develops, maintains itself and reproduces during life. This can be seen clearly in the case of populations of the nematode worm *Caenorhabditis elegans*, which is a self-fertilising hermaphrodite and therefore preserves almost complete genetic uniformity within a population of a particular strain. In spite of having a fixed genotype and being grown in a highly uniform environment, the typical laboratory population shows wide variation in the ages at death of individual adult worms (e.g., from about 10 to 30 days). In the case of humans, the consequences of intrinsic chance variations may affect fertility and life span in ways that generate positive correlation between these variables. In other words, of individuals who are fortunate in the chance factors that influence development and ageing may have above-average fertility *and* longevity.

In spite of these difficulties, we should not be daunted from investigating life history trade-offs in our species. The data available for such studies are potentially far more extensive than for any other species and the epidemiological and population genetics methodologies are well developed.

References

Cairns J (1997) Matters of life and death. Princeton University Press, Princeton.

Cummins J (1999) Evolutionary forces behind human infertility. Nature 397:557–558

Finch CE, Kirkwood TBL (2000) Chance, development and aging. Oxford University Press, New York

Gavrilov LA, Gavrilova NS (1999) Is there a reproductive cost for human longevity? J Anti-Aging Med 2:121–123

Hollingworth TH (1965) The demography of the British Peerage. Population 18(suppl):323–351

Kapahi P, Boulton ME, Kirkwood TBL (1999) Positive correlation between mammalian life spans and cellular resistance to stress. Free Radical Biol. Med. 26:495–500

Kirkwood TBL (1977) Evolution of ageing. Nature 270:301–304

Kirkwood TBL (1981) Repair and its evolution: survival versus reproduction. In: Townsend CR, Calow P (eds) Physiological ccology: an evolutionary approach to resource use. Blackwell Scientific, Oxford, pp. 165–189

Kirkwood TBL, Holliday R (1979) The evolution of ageing and longevity. Proc Roy Soc Lond B 205:531–546

Kirkwood TBL, Holliday R (1986). Ageing as a consequence of natural selection. In: Collins KJ, Bittles AH (eds) The biology of human ageing. Cambridge University Press, Cambridge, pp 1–16

Kirkwood TBL, Rose MR (1991) Evolution of senescence: late survival sacrificed for reproduction. Phil Trans Roy Soc Lond B 332:15–24

McGue M, Vaupel JW, Holm N, Harvald B (1993) Longevity is moderately heritable in a sample of Danish twins born 1870–1880. J Gerontol 48:B237–244

Miettinen O (1985) Theoretical Epidemiology. Delmar Publishers, New York

Partridge L, Barton NH (1993) Optimality, mutation and the evolution of ageing. Nature 362:305–311

Rose MR (1991) Evolutionary biology of aging. Oxford University Press, New York

Vaupel JW, Carey JR, Christensen K, Johnson TE, Yashin AI, Holm NV, Iachine IA, Kannisto V, Khazaeli AA, Liedo P. Longo VD, Zeng Y, Mantonn G, Curtsingea JW (1998) Biodemographic trajectories of longevity. Science 280:855–860

Westendorp RGJ, Kirkwood TBL (1998) Human longevity at the cost of reproductive success. Nature 396:743–746

Westendorp RGJ, Kirkwood TBL (1999a) Longevity – does family size matter? Nature 399:522

Westendorp RGJ, Kirkwood TBL (1999b) Human longevity and reproductive success: response to Gavrilov and Gavrilova. J Anti-Aging Med 2:125–126

Williams GC (1957) Pleiotropy, natural selection and the evolution of senescence. Evolution 11:398–411

Zwaan BJ, Bijlsma R, Hoekstra RF (1995) Direct selection of life span in Drosophila melanogaster. Evolution 49:649–659

Human Longevity and Parental Age at Conception

L. A. Gavrilov and N. S. Gavrilova

Abstract

Childbearing at older ages has become increasingly common in modern societies because of demographic changes (population aging), medical progress (e.g., in vitro fertilization in older women) and personal choice. Therefore, the following question has become particularly important: What will be the health and longevity of the children born to older parents? While the detriment effects of late reproduction on infant mortality and genetic diseases have been well documented, little is known about the long-term postponed effects of delayed parenting on the mortality and longevity of adult offspring. The purpose of this study is to fill the gap that exists in our knowledge about the possible postponed detrimental effects of late parenting.

Individuals born to older parents may suffer from a load of deleterious mutations. The human spontaneous mutation rate for DNA base substitutions is reported to be very high, presumably more than one new mutation per zygote (Crow 1997). The mutation rate is much higher in male sperm cells than in female ovaries and increases with paternal age due to the large number of cell divisions in the male germ line (Crow 1997). In this study we checked whether human longevity is affected by the increased mutation load expected for the progeny of older fathers. For this purpose the high quality data (more than 15,000 records) on European royal and noble families were collected, computerized and analyzed. The data on offspring life span were adjusted for historical trends and fluctuations in life expectancy of human birth cohorts. Also, to avoid bias in estimating the offspring life span, only extinct cohorts were analyzed (born in 1800–1899).

We found (after controlling for maternal age at reproduction, paternal and maternal longevity and sex-specific cohort life expectancy) that adult daughters (30+ years) born to older fathers (45–55 years) lived shorter lives, and for each additional year of paternal age the daughters lost about 0.5 ± 0.2 years of their life span. In contrast to daughters, the sons were not significantly affected by delayed paternal parenting. This result was also confirmed after taking into account additional confounding variables (nationality, birth order, cause of death and loss of parents before age 20) using multiple regression on nominal variables. Since only daughters inherit the paternal X chromosome, this sex-specific life span shortening for daughters born to older fathers might indicate that the

Robine et al. (Eds.)
Sex and Longevity: Sexuality, Gender,
Reproduction, Parenthood
© Springer-Verlag Berlin Heidelberg 2000

genes affecting longevity and sensitive to mutation load are probably concentrated in the X chromosome.

The mutation theory of life span predicts that those individuals who have a low mutation rate in their somatic and germ cells will live longer lives and will be able to produce normal offspring even in old age. This prediction was tested in this study for the first time and proved to be correct. Daughters born to old fathers lived shorter lives but those daughters who were born to longer-lived fathers (81+ years) were not affected by the late paternal age at conception.

Another new finding of this study is that daughters born to particularly young fathers (below 25 years) also tended to live shorter lives. This finding is consistent with existing epidemiological data on the increased risk of congenital diseases and impaired behavioral performance among children born to particularly young fathers, as well as with similar animal studies. Thus, the age constraints for the donors of sperm cells (used for in vitro fertilization) should be carefully revised.

Why Studies of Parental-Age Effects Are so Important

Practical Importance of the Studies

Childbearing at older ages has become increasingly common in modern societies because of demographic changes (population aging), medical progress [e.g., in vitro fertilization (IVF) in older women] and personal choice (Kuliev and Modell 1990). For example, in the United States the number of births to older mothers (35–39 years and 40+ years) more than doubled since 1980, whereas the number of births to younger mothers (below age 30) did not increase (see Table 1).

Birth rates for older fathers (ages 45–49 and 50–54) are also increasing (US Monthly Vital Statistics Report 1997), and this trend may even accelerate in the future due to medical progress (Viagra, for example). Moreover, it has become possible to enjoy fatherhood at an older age through an assisted reproduction technique called intracytoplasmic sperm injection (ICSI). A few spermatozoa are

Table 1. American mothers are becoming older. Increasing number of births to older mothers

| Age of mother | Total number of births in thousands in the United States, by year | | | | | | | | | | |
	1980	1985	1986	1987	1988	1989	1990	1991	1992	1993	1994
<20	562	478	472	473	489	518	533	532	518	501	518
20–24	1,226	1,141	1,102	1,076	1,067	1,078	1,094	1,090	1,070	1,038	1,001
25–29	1,108	1,201	1,200	1,216	1,239	1,263	1,277	1,220	1,179	1,129	1,089
30–34	550	696	721	761	804	842	886	885	895	901	906
35–39	141	214	230	248	270	294	318	331	345	357	372
40 and more	24	29	31	36	41	46	50	54	58	61	66

Source: US Bureau of the Census (1997)

extracted either from the semen or testis of old men, and each sperm is then injected into an individual egg that is implanted in the fallopian tube. Thus, old age and even clinical death are not obstacles to fatherhood any longer.

However, one important concern remains: What will be the health and longevity of the children born to older parents? While the detrimental effects of late reproduction on infant mortality and genetic diseases have been well documented (see below), little is known about the long-term postponed effects of delayed parenting on the mortality and longevity of adult offspring. The purpose of this study is to fill the gap that exists in our knowledge about the possible postponed detrimental effects of late parenting.

Scientific Significance of Studies of Parental-Age Effects

Despite their practical and scientific importance, the fundamental mechanisms that determine human longevity are still unknown. In particular, it is not yet known whether genomic damage is the most critically important force influencing human longevity (mutation theory of aging; see Vijg and Gossen 1993). One approach to resolving this problem is to study the life span of offspring born to parents at different ages and to determine whether the established, age-related accumulation of the DNA damage in parental germ cells is important for the longevity of the offspring. The scientific credibility of such an approach is supported by the recent findings that paternal age at reproduction is the major determinant of the level of mutation load in humans (Crow 1993, 1995, 1997).

According to existing evidence, parental age has many detrimental influences on the longevity of offspring (for an exhaustive review of this topic, see Finch 1990). The major maternal age-related changes in humans are increases in fetal aneuploidy later in reproductive life such as:

- Down's syndrome (trisomy 21) (Hook 1986; Carothers et al. 1978; Bocciolone et al. 1989; Erickson 1978; Saxen 1983)
- Klinefelter's syndrome (XXY) (Carothers et al. 1978; Carothers and Filippi 1988)
- Edward's syndrome (trisomy 18) and Patau's syndrome (trisomy 13) (Hook 1986; Carothers et al. 1978).

Advanced maternal age also remains an important independent risk factor for fetal death (Parazzini et al. 1990; Resseguie 1976; Fretts et al. 1995).

The detrimental effect of late paternal reproduction is also well known: advanced paternal age has been associated with an increase in new dominant mutations in offspring that result in congenital anomalies (Auroux 1993a, b, 1983; Risch et al. 1987; Lian et al. 1986; McIntosh et al. 1995; Meacham and Murray 1994; Savitz et al. 1991; Friedman 1981; Bordson and Leonardo 1991; Vogel 1983; Carothers et al. 1986; Young et al. 1987). In particular, paternal age is responsible for new dominant autosomal mutations that cause different malformations, including:

- achondroplasia (Auroux 1993a, b; Lian et al. 1986)
- Apert syndrome (Auroux 1993a, b)
- Marfan syndrome (Auroux 1993a, b)
- osteogenesis imperfecta (Carothers et al. 1986; Young et al. 1987) and other inherited diseases.

Older paternal age was observed among patients with Costello syndrome (Lurie 1994), chondrodysplasia punctata (Sheffield et al. 1976), fibrodysplasia ossificans progressiva (Connor and Evans 1982; Rogers and Chase 1979), and thanatophoric displasia (Martinez-Frias et al. 1988). Advanced paternal age at reproduction is also associated with increased risk of preauricular cyst, nasal aplasia, cleft palate, hydrocephalus, pulmonic stenosis, urethral stenosis, and hemangioma (Savitz et al. 1991). Increased paternal age at childbirth is also an important independent risk factor for neonatal and infant mortality (Gourbin and Wunsch 1999).

There is, however, one very important question that has yet to be addressed: does parental age at birth (or conception) influence the longevity of the vast majority of the population of so-called "normal healthy people" who do not suffer from aneuploidy and other obvious genetic conditions that tend to appear early in life? In other words, are aging-related diseases associated with paternal and maternal age at conception or birth? It is possible to address this question by examining the life expectancy of adults (say, at age 30 and older) as a function of parental age at reproduction. By adult age a substantial portion of the subpopulation suffering from early-acting deleterious mutations has already died (i.e., selected out). The information on potential life-shortening effects of late parental reproduction on adult offspring is notable because it addresses a possibly important gap in knowledge about the mechanisms of human longevity, the aging process itself, and of the possible role of accumulated genetic damage in the germ line on aging and longevity.

Historical Background

The first mention in the historical literature suggesting a possible life-shortening effect on offspring of delayed parenting was made by the French naturalist Buffon (1826), who noted that when old men procreate "they often engender monsters, deformed children, still more defective than their father" (see Robine and Allard 1997).

Later, intensive studies of human genealogical data were initiated by Karl Pearson (Beeton and Pearson 1901) and Raymond Pearl (Pearl 1931; Pearl and Dewitt 1934) and developed further by other researchers (Hawkins et al. 1965; Abbott et al. 1974; Murphy 1978; Wyshak 1978; Desjardins and Charbonneau 1990; Bocquet-Appel and Jakobi 1991). However, these empirical studies were focused specifically on inheritance of human longevity rather than on the question of parental age effects at birth on offspring longevity, as proposed here.

Before our early preliminary studies on this topic (Gavrilov et al. 1995a, b), other researchers partially addressed the same issue (Jalavisto 1950; Philippe

1980). Jalavisto (1950) analyzed 12,786 published family records of the Finnish and Swedish middle class and nobility born in 1500–1829. Unfortunately, in this interesting study the secular changes in human life span during this long historical period (1500–1829) were not taken into account, and the investigator did not attempt to control for the possible effects of other confounding factors. Jalavisto (1950) concluded that offspring born to older mothers live significantly shorter lives, and the age of the father was of no importance. These observations deserve to be replicated in future studies by controlling for the effects of other confounding factors and historical changes in the life expectancy of birth cohorts.

In 1980 Pierre Philippe studied five birth cohorts (1800-29, 1830–49, 1850–69, 1870–79, 1880–99) from a small rural population of Isle-aux-Coudres, Quebec, Canada. Multiple discriminant analysis was used to study the effects of different familial characteristics (such as parental consanguinity, maternal and paternal age at time of childbirth, birth order, the interval since the previous birth, months of birth, viability of the preceding infant, etc.) on offspring age at death, broken into 10 age groups (from age 0 through 90 years and over). Surprisingly, possibly the most evident and important predictors of offspring longevity (paternal and maternal life spans) were not included in the analysis. Also, the author noted the following: "taking into consideration the possibility of differential emigration" from this small rural area (Isle-aux-Coudres), the results of analysis "must certainly be regarded cautiously" (Philippe 1980, p. 215). Indeed, in many cases the results of this analysis were not statistically significant, perhaps because of the small size of the birth cohorts (105–298 cases only in each cohort), and also because of possible overloading of the analysis by too many variables (up to 26 binary variables were included in the analysis). In spite of these problems, the author of this study made an intriguing observation that increased maternal age at time of childbirth (35 years and above) is the main factor common to both early (0–5 years) and late (70 years and above) death (Philippe 1980). By contrast, increased father's age was uncommon for long-lived offspring (Philippe 1980).

These important and contradictory observations deserve to be tested in future studies by using larger sample sizes and controlling for parental longevity. Control for parental longevity is important since recent studies have demonstrated that among long-lived women the proportion of those able to become mothers after 40 years is four times higher compared to "normal" women (Perls et al. 1997). Thus, increased offspring longevity might not be due to the older age of mother at childbirth per se, but due to higher longevity of such mothers and the inheritance of the longevity by the offspring. This hypothesis deserves to be tested in future studies.

Recent Preliminary Studies

Our first preliminary studies on long-term effects of parental age at reproduction on offspring longevity in humans were based on the statistical analysis of human genealogical data on European royal and noble families. We demonstrated that paternal age at reproduction has a specific threshold life-shortening effect on daughters rather than on sons (Gavrilov et al. 1995a, b, 1997a–c; Gavrilov and Gavrilova 1997a, b). Attempts to reproduce these results were made recently by other authors (Robine and Allard 1997) using archives in Arles, France, but in this study both sexes (daughters and sons) were mixed and analyzed together, so the results are not comparable. Since paternal and maternal ages at reproduction are correlated (older mothers tend to have older spouses), it is important to study the effect of maternal age on offspring longevity. It was found that for mothers in the reproductive age range of 20–39 there was no observed effect of maternal age on the longevity of adult children (Gavrilov et al. 1997b). Since the reproductive life span of females is shorter than in males because of menopause, the sample size for children of very old mothers (more than 40 years old) has so far been too small to draw any conclusions on this issue. Further studies designed to increase sample sizes are therefore important in order to assess the independent effects of both paternal and maternal ages at reproduction on offspring longevity.

Biological Ideas Related to Studies of Parental Age Effects

Two preliminary observations were made in the above-mentioned studies (Gavrilov et al. 1995a, b, 1997a, c; Gavrilov and Gavrilova 1997a, b).

First, the effect of parental reproductive age on longevity of adult children was observed for fathers only (specific paternal effect).

Second, paternal age is detrimental for longevity of daughters only (specific sex-linked effect on daughters).

Both observations may have biological explanations. It has already been established that the mutation rate in human paternal germ cells is much higher than in maternal ones (Crow 1993, 1995, 1997), with the age of the father demonstrated to be the main factor determining the spontaneous mutation rate of nuclear DNA (Crow 1993, 1995, 1997). Thus, there is good reason to expect the presence of a paternal rather than a maternal influence on offspring longevity, since mutational load in germ cells is mainly of paternal origin. The reason for this specific paternal effect is that the mutation rate is largely determined by the number of cell divisions and DNA replications, a time when errors are introduced into the DNA of the germ cells. Since the number of cell divisions between zygote and sperm (in males) is much larger than between zygote and egg (in females), much higher accumulation of DNA damage in paternal germ cells should be expected. In humans, the estimated number of cell divisions in females between zygote and egg is 24, which is largely independent of age (Vogel and Motulsky 1997). In males the number of cell divisions between zygote and sperm is much larger. The number of divisions prior to a sperm produced at puberty (e.g., age 13) is estimated at 36, and thereafter the number increases by 23 divisions per year (Vogel and Motulsky 1997). So, at age 20 the number of cell divisions is about 200 and has increased by age 50 to about 890 cell divisions Thus, there is reason to hypothesize specific paternal effects on mutational load and longevity in the offspring.

The second observation from our previous work is that high paternal reproductive age is detrimental for daughters only. Since the paternal X chromosome is inherited by daughters rather than sons, this observation might indicate that critical genes (critical targets for mutational damage) important for longevity are located on the X chromosome. This suggested explanation is valid for both dominant and recessive mutations, since only one X chromosome is active in each particular human female cell and the second X chromosome is inactivated after the first 48 hours of the zygote's development.

It is important to note that there is a good evolutionary reason for mother Nature to hide critical genes on the X chromosome, since it is one of the safest locations in the human genome. The reason is that the level of DNA damage in a particular chromosome is determined by its exposure to the "male environment." For example, the most unfavorable situation is observed for Y chromosomes that are male-specific. Since the Y chromosome is always in males whereas an autosome is in males only half of the time, the level of DNA damage for this chromosome should be especially high. Indeed, it has already been demonstrated that the primate evolution rates (that are correlated to mutation rates) of the Y-linked argininosuccinate synthetase pseudogene are about two times higher than those of its autosomal counterpart (Miyata et al. 1990). Thus, in a sense the Y chromosome is the most "dangerous" place in the human genome, which might be the reason why so few genes are associated with that chromosome. Contrary to the Y chromosome, the X chromosome is less exposed to the "male environment" since females have two copies of it whereas males have only one copy. Since one-third of all human X chromosomes are in males, the X chromosome should have a mutation rate that is two-thirds that of the autosomes ($2/3 = 0.67$). Miyata et al. (1990) demonstrated that the X/autosome ratio for silent changes in DNA during primate evolution (that is proportional to mutation rates) is in fact 0.69 (very close to the expected 0.67 ratio).

Recent studies on rodents have also demonstrated that the rate of substitution of synonymous mutations in X-linked genes to that in autosomal ones is 0.62 ± 0.04, which is consistent with X-linked genes having a reduced mutation rate (McVean and Hurst 1997). Thus, the X chromosome is in a sense the "safest" place in the human genome, implying that there is a good evolutionary reason to hide the most critical genes in this particular chromosome. One such critical gene located in the X chromosome is the gene for DNA polymerase alpha, an enzyme involved in DNA replication (Wang et al. 1985). Mutations of this critical enzyme may result in a decrease in the accuracy of DNA replication and thus a catastrophic increase in mutation rates (Orgel 1963, 1970). Other critical genes located on the X chromosome are genes for glucose-6-phosphate dehydrogenase (important for protection against oxidative damage of DNA and other structures) and plasma membrane Ca^{++} transporting ATPase.

Another possible explanation for the critical importance of mutation load on the X chromosome is related to the special status of this chromosome in females. As already noted, in each particular female cell only one X chromosome is active, and the second one is inactivated. Thus, at the intracellular level there is no genetic redundancy for genes located on the X chromosome compared to genes located on autosomes (two active copies are there). For this reason, deleterious recessive mutations could be completely complemented if they are heterozygous and are located in autosomes, but they **cannot** be complemented at the intracellular level if they are located on the X chromosome. Complementation of these mutations is possible at the intercellular level only. Mutations on X chromosomes may therefore be more "visible" through their effects on mortality compared to mutations on other chromosomes.

The specific, life-shortening effect of paternal age on daughters' longevity might also be caused by the specific increase of mutation rates on the paternal X chromosome. The X is methylated in the male germ line and for this reason should be more prone to mutations than maternal X, as both X chromosomes are unmethylated in the female germ line (Driscoll and Migeon 1990).

The X chromosome hypothesis provides a very specific prediction that we propose to test in future studies. Since the grandfather's X chromosome is inherited through the mother's side only, one might expect a specific effect of the reproductive age of the maternal grandfather. Specifically, this hypothesis predicts that grandchildren (grandsons in particular) should live shorter lives if their mother was born to an older grandfather (Gavrilov and Gavrilova 1997a). This specific age effect of the maternal grandfather has already been demonstrated for some X-linked genetic diseases, such as Duchenne muscular dystrophy (caused by mutation in locus on Xp21; Bucher et al. 1980), hemophilia A and Lesch-Nyhan disease (reviewed by Vogel and Motulsky 1997). However, this hypothesis has never been tested for the duration of human life; we plan to test it in our future studies.

Possible Implications from Studies of Parental-Age Effects

The following important implications may be expected from future studies of parental age effects on offspring longevity:

1) If future studies confirm significant parental age effects in humans, these findings will have a profound effect on the concepts and methods of genetic, epidemiologic longevity studies. In particular, all previous epidemiological and genetic studies of human aging and life span will have to be revised, controlling for the confounding effects of the parental age variables.

2) Physicians will become aware whether potential patients born to older parents represent a risk group that should be screened more carefully for health problems at older ages. For example, it was recently found that older paternal age is a risk factor for a sporadic form of Alzheimer's disease, whereas maternal age has no prognostic importance (Bertram et al. 1998). If parental age effects prove to be as important as the effects of smoking habits, the implications for life insurance practice could become obvious.

3) Potential older parents (and physicians involved in new reproductive technologies) will receive important new knowledge about health risks associated

with parenting in later life. In the case of IVF, the age constraints for donors of sperm and ova cells will be more carefully considered.

4) On the other hand, if parental age effects prove to be insignificant in future studies, this would be a great relief for older parents and their children. This is a particularly relevant issue today given trends in delaying childbearing in the United States and other developed nations. This outcome of the study will also become a scientific challenge for biologists, who have to explain how the human species manages to cope with high mutation rates. This problem has already received increasing attention from the scientific community (see recent discussions on this problem in scientific literature; Crow 1997, 1999; Eyre-Walker and Keightley 1999; Gavrilov and Gavrilova 1999a).

Research Findings and Discussion

The First Wave of Exploratory Studies: Analysis of Cross-Tabulations

In our first study of parental age effects for 8,518 persons from European aristocratic families with well-known genealogy (Van Hueck 1977–1997; Gavrilova and Gavrilov 1999), we found a strong inverse relationship between father's age at reproduction and daughter's (not son's) longevity (Gavrilov and Gavrilova 1997a; Gavrilov et al. 1997a). The results of this study are summarized in Table 2.

Note that daughters born to old fathers lose about 4.4 years of their life and these losses are statistically significant ($p < 0.01$; Student's test, $t = 3.1$), whereas sons are not significantly affected. This finding is in accord with the mutation theory of aging (Vijg and Gossen 1993), since paternal age at reproduction is

Table 2. Human longevity and sex differential in longevity as a function of father's age at reproduction

| Paternal age at reproduction[a] (years) | Mean age at death[b] ± standard error (years) | | Sex differential in life span (years) |
	Daughters (sample size)	Sons (sample size)	
20–29	66.5 ± 0.7 (592)	61.3 ± 0.4 (1,238)	5.2 ± 0.8
30–39	65.9 ± 0.5 (1,214)	60.8 ± 0.3 (2,580)	5.1 ± 0.6
40–49	64.4 ± 0.7 (694)	60.5 ± 0.4 (1,543)	3.9 ± 0.8
50–59	62.1 ± 1.2 (206)	60.3 ± 0.7 (451)	1.8 ± 1.4

[a] Data are controlled for father's longevity (all fathers lived 50 years and more) to eliminate bias caused by correlation between father's and offspring life span.

[b] Human longevity was calculated for adults (those who survived to age 30) born in the 18th and 19th centuries. The data for those born in the 20th century were excluded from the analysis to have unbiased estimates of longevity for extinct birth cohorts.

considered to be the main factor determining human spontaneous mutation rate (Crow 1993, 1995, 1997). Also, since only daughters inherit the paternal X chromosome, this sex-specific decrease in longevity of daughters born to old fathers might indicate that human longevity genes (crucial, housekeeping genes) sensitive to mutational load might be located in this chromosome (Gavrilov and Gavrilova 1997a; Gavrilov et al. 1997a).

Another interesting observation is that sex differences in human longevity are a function of paternal age at reproduction. The data presented in Table 2 show that females live longer than males when fathers are young, whereas in the case of old fathers sex differences are very small and statistically insignificant (Gavrilova et al. 1995; Gavrilov et al. 1995b, 1997a). This preliminary observation may also have a biological explanation. Since females have two X chromosomes, they are genetically more redundant than males, who have only one X chromosome. However, when the father is older and the X chromosome transferred to his daughter has a higher mutational load, there is no longer a difference in genetic redundancy between males and females, since both have only one intact (maternal) X chromosome. Thus, there is every reason to expect that with increases in paternal reproductive age the sex differences in offspring longevity should decrease (see Table 2, the column for the sex differential in longevity, supporting this hypothesis).

It should be noted, however, that in these first studies (Gavrilov and Gavrilova 1997a; Gavrilov et al. 1997a) some possibly important covariates and confounding factors were not controlled for, such as maternal age at reproduction (which is strongly correlated with paternal age), historical trends and fluctuations in life expectancy of birth cohorts, and parental longevity (age at death). Thus, the next logical step in this line of inquiry is to fill this gap and examine the previous observations on the life-shortening effects of late paternal reproduction, taking into account the other important covariates mentioned above.

The Second Wave of Exploratory Studies: Multiple Linear Regression

In this next step of our study we increased the sample size and re-analyzed the data for the offspring born to older fathers at age 35–55. Offspring life span was analyzed for adults (those who survived by age 30) to study the long-term, postponed effects of late reproduction of the parents. The data for offspring born in the 20th century were excluded from the analysis in order to have unbiased estimates of longevity for extinct birth cohorts. The data for offspring born before the 19th century were also excluded in order to minimize the heterogeneity of the sample.

For each birth cohort the mean sex-specific expectation of life at age 30 was calculated and used as an independent variable in a multiple linear regression model to control for cohort and secular trends and fluctuations in human longevity. Offspring longevity for each particular sex (4,566 records for males and 2,068 records for females) was considered as a dependent variable in the multiple

Table 3. Parental predictors of human longevity. Coefficients (slopes) of multiple linear regression ± standard error

Variable	Sons	Daughters
Paternal age at reproduction	−0.06 ± 0.05	**−0.16 ± 0.07**
Maternal age at reproduction	0.03 ± 0.04	0.02 ± 0.06
Paternal age at death	0.13 ± 0.02	0.09 ± 0.03
Maternal age at death	0.03 ± 0.01	0.04 ± 0.02
Cohort life expectancy	1.07 ± 0.10	1.04 ± 0.05
Other characteristics of regression		
Sample size	4,566	2,068
Multiple R	0.2	0.4
F ratio	37.2	86.3

regression model (program 1R in BMDP statistical package) and a function of five independent predictors: paternal age at reproduction in the range of 35–55 years (where the life-shortening effect was previously detected; Gavrilov and Gavrilova 1997b), maternal age at reproduction (control for maternal age is important since it is correlated with paternal age), paternal age at death, maternal age at death (to control for heritability of human longevity), and sex-specific cohort life expectancy (control for cohort and secular trends and fluctuations).

The results of this study are presented in Table 3. The regression slope (b) for daughter's longevity as a function of paternal age at reproduction is negative (b = −0.16 ± 0.07) and this inverse relationship is statistically significant (Student test, t = −2.35, P = 0.02) even when the effects of the other important four covariates are taken into account. In the case of sons the association with paternal age at reproduction is much weaker (regression slope, b = −0.06 ± 0.05) and statistically insignificant (Student test, t = −1.20, P = 0.23).

Thus, this study lends support to the previous preliminary observations (Gavrilov and Gavrilova 1997a; Gavrilov et al. 1995b, 1997a) on the sex-specific, life-shortening effect of late paternal reproduction on daughters' longevity. It would be interesting to continue these studies and to check the prediction of the X chromosome hypothesis: the expected specific life-shortening effect of late grandpaternal reproduction from the mother's side only.

The results described above were based on the assumption that the dependence between offspring longevity and paternal age at reproduction could be considered approximately linear for paternal ages in the range of 35–55 years. The next step of the study was to check whether this assumption was valid. For this reason we re-analyzed the data for different ranges of paternal age at reproduction. It turned out that for the subgroup of younger fathers (35–45 years), the mean loss of daughters' life span is very small (0.02 ± 0.12 years lost per each additional year of paternal age) and statistically insignificant (sample size, n = 1651; Student test, t = 0.16; p = 0.87), whereas for older fathers (45–55 years) this loss is particularly high (0.48 ± 0.21 years lost per each additional year of paternal age) and statistically significant (n = 598; t = 2.34; p = 0.02). These results are consistent with the general conclusion of Professor James Crow on the non-linear accelerating increase of mutation rates with paternal age (Crow 1993, 1995, 1997).

One possible explanation for this threshold effect of paternal age might be the competition among sperm cells. Since only one of a huge number of sperm cells succeeds in fertilization in each particular case, damaged sperm cells with a high mutational load may not withstand this strong competition. Only at very old ages, when the proportion of damaged sperm cells becomes higher than some threshold level, does the selection mechanism finally fail and accumulation of mutational load becomes evident (Gavrilov et al. 1997a).

There may be another explanation for the threshold nature of paternal effect on offspring longevity. Since short-lived fathers can participate in reproduction at young ages only, the detrimental effect of age-related accumulation of muta-tional load in paternal germ cells might be compensated for by selection effects (i.e., the population of old fathers is also the population of survivors compared to young fathers). In other words, the threshold behavior might be an artifact caused by the heterogeneity of the population. It is therefore important to study the effect of paternal age on a more homogeneous population of longer-lived fathers.

The results of our cohort study of the genealogical records of 8,518 persons from European aristocratic families presented in Table 2 have shown that the life-shortening effect of paternal age is more gradual (as opposed to operating under a threshold) if it is studied in a relatively homogeneous population of long-lived fathers (with life span of more than 50 years; Gavrilov et al. 1997a). This conclu-sion might be of practical importance since the effect of paternal age is not restricted by relatively rare cases of old fathers (50 years and above) but might be important in developed nations where a significantly larger portion of offspring are likely to be born to middle-aged fathers.

It is important to continue these studies to try to resolve the controversy between threshold and gradual parental age effects observed in different types of data analysis.

The Third Wave of Exploratory Studies: Analysis of Contour Maps for Life span

In this next stage of our study we increased the sample size (up to 17,215 comput-erized genealogical records) and applied the methods of contour maps to study parental age effects on offspring life span.

The idea behind this method is quite simple: the levels of life span are mapped in a way similar to the mapping of surface altitude in geographical maps. The horizontal, X axis corresponds to paternal age at childbirth (20–60 years), similar to the "West-East" dimension used in geographical maps. The vertical, Y axis corresponds to the maternal age at childbirth (15–45 years), similar to the "South-North" dimension used in geographical maps. Data for each person are plotted as points with X and Y coordinates corresponding to paternal and mater-nal ages when the person was born. The third dimension in this map is the per-

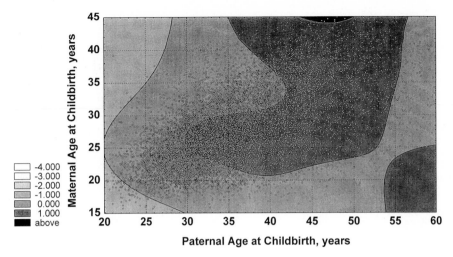

Fig. 1. Contour plot for levels of sons' life span (deviation from cohort mean) as a function of paternal (X axis) and maternal (Y axis) ages at childbirth. European noble families: 1800–1880 birth cohorts. Spline smooth. 12,015 cases

son's life span (expressed in normalized form as a deviation from control level: the mean life span of persons of the same sex, born in the same calendar year).

These life span residuals form the surface that is some years above or below the control life span level (similar to the sea level used in geographical maps). The surface is colored, like in geographical maps, depending on the direction and the extent of the deviation from the control life span level. In our study we used white for the lowest level of life span, grays of different intensities for intermediate life span levels and black for the highest level of life span.

As a result of such data presentation, contour life span maps are produced that allow one to visualize the large amounts of data in the form of colored contours. The data for men (sons) and women (daughters) are analyzed separately, producing two different maps (Fig. 1 and 2) with the same scales to allow their comparison.

The contour life span map for sons (Fig. 1) supports our previous findings that neither the father's nor the mother's age at childbirth has a significant effect on the son's life span. The whole map area is covered by intermediate grays, which indicate a very flat landscape ("life span prairie") and nothing interesting to study.

In contrast, the contour life span map for daughters (Fig. 2) has a very interesting and contrasting landscape ("life span precipice"). The lowest levels of daughters' life span (white areas) are observed for daughters born to young mothers (15–20 years) and to fathers of extreme ages (either below 25 years or above 55 years). In these two extreme cases the daughters' life span is three to four years below the reference level.

The highest levels of daughters' life span (black area) are observed for daughters born to older mothers (above 30–35 years) and middle-aged fathers (35–45

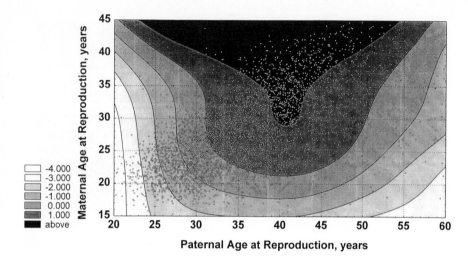

Fig. 2. Contour plot for levels of daughters' life span (deviation from cohort mean) as a function of paternal (X axis) and maternal (Y axis) ages at childbirth. European noble families: 1800–1880 birth cohorts. Spline smooth. 5,200 cases

years). In this case the daughters' life span is more than one year above the reference life span level. The black area observed for daughters of younger fathers ("Northwestern" part of the map; Fig. 2) should not be considered seriously, since there are no real data there (no couples composed of 20–30-year-old fathers and 40- to 45-year-old mothers).

If one fixes the mother's age at some level (say, age 30) and studies the paternal age effect (moving horizontally from the "West" to the "East"; Fig. 2), the daughters' life span first increases, reaching the maximum at a paternal age of 40–45 years. After that age the daughters' life span starts to decline. The decline in life span of daughters born to older fathers (above 40–45 years) is consistent with our previous findings (see earlier). However, the paradoxical increase in daughters' life span with paternal age for younger fathers (20–40 years) is a new finding that deserves to be studied in more detail.

One possible explanation of the "young father-short daughters' life span" paradox is that short-lived fathers cannot be old! Thus, the proportion of short-lived fathers with genetic diseases should be higher among younger fathers. Since human life span is heritable (Gavrilova et al. 1998), this may explain the observed paradox.

To test this hypothesis, we studied the contour life span maps, where the paternal life span variable is included in the analysis (Fig. 3–4). In these maps the horizontal, X axis corresponds to paternal life span (40–95 years, "West-East" dimension). The vertical, Y axis corresponds to paternal age at childbirth (20–60 years, "South-North" dimension). The maps for sons (Fig. 3) and daughters (Fig. 4) have the same scale of gradations and colors, allowing their comparison.

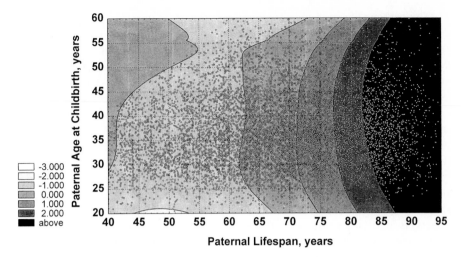

Fig. 3. Contour plot for levels of sons' life span (deviation from cohort mean) as a function of paternal life span (X axis) and age at childbirth (Y axis). European noble families: 1800–1880 birth cohorts. Spline smooth. 12,015 cases

The contour life span map for sons (Fig. 3) has vertical orientation of isolines, with the highest life span levels in the right, "Eastern" part of the map, corresponding to long-lived fathers (85–95 years). This pattern ("life span uphill") is consistent with our prior knowledge that sons' life span is determined by fathers' life span and does not depend on fathers' age at childbirth (no "South-North" differences).

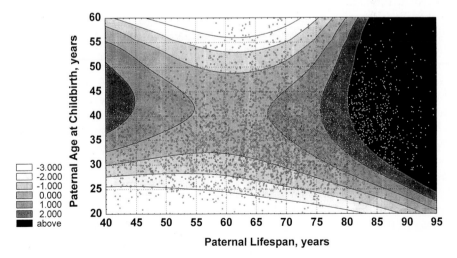

Fig. 4. Contour plot for levels of daughters' life span (deviation from cohort mean) as a function of paternal life span (X axis) and age at childbirth (Y axis). European noble families: 1800–1880 birth cohorts. Spline smooth. 5,200 cases

The contour life span map for daughters (Fig. 4) is particularly interesting: it looks like a "life span col." In addition to the paternal life span effects ("West-East" differences) there is also an effect of paternal age at childbirth ("South-North" differences). What is important is that, at any level of paternal life span, there is an optimal level of paternal age at childbirth (35–45 years), where daughters have the highest life span (horizontal "West-East life span ridge").

Thus, the shorter life span of the daughters born to particularly young fathers (20–25 years) is not an artifact caused by the shorter life span of young fathers. In fact, the phenomenon of short life span of early daughters is observed at any level of paternal life span (see the bottom of Fig. 4).

Analysis of the scientific literature suggests that there may be a fundamental biological explanation of the "young father – short daughters' life span" paradox. The risk of congenital heart defects (ventricular septal defects and atrial septal defects) is increased among the offspring of older fathers (over 35 years) and also among the offspring of particularly young fathers (under 20 years; Olshan et al. 1994). Children born to younger fathers (under 20 years) have increased risk of neural tube defects, hypospadias, cystic kidney, and Down syndrome (McIntosh et al. 1995).

In the mouse, offspring born to mature fathers exhibit better behavioral performances (for spontaneous activity in both sexes and learning capacity in males) than those born to particularly young, post-pubescent fathers (Auroux et al. 1998). Similar results were obtained for humans in a study that involved the distribution of scores obtained in psychometric tests by 18-year-old male subjects, according to their father's age at the time of their birth. This distribution indicated not only that increased paternal age is accompanied by effects similar to those observed in animals, but also that very young paternal age was also related to these effects. Thus, the curve of such scores produced an inverted U-shape, with maximum scores obtained when the father was about 30 years of age. Maternal age did not appear to play a part in this event. These results pose the problem of identifying genetic and/or psychosocial factors that might have an impact on the quality of the conceptus (Auroux et al. 1989).

The practical importance of these findings is obvious: the age constraints for the donors of sperm cells in IVF should probably be revised to exclude not only the old donors but also those donors who are too young (under 25 years).

Another interesting observation that comes from the analysis of the data in Figure 4 (large black spot in the "North-Eastern" part of the map) is that longer-lived fathers (over 80–85 years) produce longer-lived daughters, even when they are old (55–60 years). In other words, daughters born to older fathers live shorter lives only in those cases when their fathers die before the age of 80–85 years. The importance of this finding and its possible explanation are discussed in the next section of this chapter.

Coming to Understand the Parental Age Effects on Human Life span

In this final stage of data analysis we applied a multiple regression analysis with nominal variables, which is a very flexible tool to control for effects of both quantitative and qualitative (categorized) variables. This method also allows one to accommodate for complex non-linear and non-monotonic effects of predictor variables. We used the data for extinct birth cohorts (born in 1800–1880) free of censored observations and tested a long list of explanatory and potentially confounding variables (see below) to consider all possible artifacts.

Life span of adult (30+) progeny (sons and daughters separately) was considered as a dependent outcome variable in multivariate regression with dummy (0–1) variables using a SPSS statistical package. The independent predictor variables included 12 types of binary variables:

1) calendar year of birth (to control for historical increase in life expectancy as well as for complex secular fluctuations in life span). The whole birth year period of 1800–1880 was split into five-year intervals (16 intervals) presented by 15 binary (0–1) variables with the reference level set at 1875–1880 birth years.

2) maternal life span (to control for maternal influence through combined genetic effects and shared environment). The maternal life span data were grouped into five-year intervals (15 intervals) with the exception of the first (15–29 years) and the last (95–110 years) longer intervals with small numbers of observations. The data were coded with 14 dummy variables with the reference level set at 75–80 years for maternal life span.

3) paternal life span (to control for paternal influence through combined genetic effects and shared environment). The data were grouped and coded in a way similar to maternal life span (see above).

4) maternal age when a person (proband) was born. This is the key explanatory variable to study maternal age effects on offspring life span. The data for mother's age were grouped in five-year intervals (seven intervals to cover the age range of 15–60 years) with the exception of the last, longer interval of 45–59 years with small numbers of observations. Maternal age of 25–29 years was selected as a reference.

5) father's age when a person was born. This is the key explanatory variable to study paternal age effects on offspring life span. The data were grouped and coded in five-year intervals (nine intervals to cover the age range of 15–80 years) with the exception of the first (15–24 years) and the last (60–79 years) longer intervals with small numbers of observations. Paternal age of 40–44 years was selected as a reference.

6) birth order. This variable is represented by binary variable coded as 1 when the individual was a first born child and coded as 0 otherwise.

7) nationality. The nationality of the individual is represented by a set of four categories – Germans, British, Russians and others. Germans (the largest group in our sample) is selected as a reference group.

8) cause of death (violent versus non-violent). This variable is represented as a set of four dummy variables: 1) violent cause of death (war losses, accidents,

etc.), 2) death in prison and other unfavorable conditions (concentration camp, etc.), 3) death from acute infections (cholera, etc.) and 4) maternal death (for women only). Deaths from all other causes combined were considered as a reference outcome.

9) loss of the father in the formative years of life (before age 20). This is a binary variable coded as 1 when father was lost before the age of 20 and coded as 0 otherwise.

10) loss of the mother before age 20. This binary variable is coded as 1 in those cases when mother was lost before the age of 20 and coded as 0 otherwise.

11) loss of both parents (orphanhood) before the age of 20. This binary variable is coded as 1 in those cases when both parents were lost before the age of 20 and coded as 0 otherwise.

12) month of birth. This variable was included in the analysis because previous studies have found that month of birth is an important predictor of adult life span (Gavrilov and Gavrilova 1999b; Doblhammer 1999), particularly for daughters (Gavrilov and Gavrilova 1999b). This variable was represented as a set of 11 dummy variables, with those born in August considered as a reference group.

The results of data analysis are presented in Figures 5–10. Figure 5 depicts the net (adjusted) effects of paternal age at reproduction on daughters' life span when the effects of other variables (listed above) are controlled for. Daughters born to older fathers (55–59 years, 72 cases) live shorter lives compared to daughters born to middle-aged fathers (40–44 years): a difference in life expectancy at adult ages (30+) is 4.52 ± 1.94 years, which is statistically significant (t-ratio = −2.33, p = 0.02).

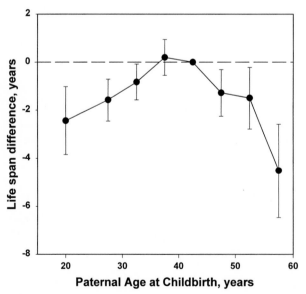

Fig. 5. Effect of paternal age at childbirth on daughters' life span based on 4,369 daughters from European aristocratic families born from 1800–1880. Life expectancy of adult women (30+) as a function of father's age when these women were born (expressed as a difference from the reference level for those born to fathers aged 40–44 years). The data are point estimates (with standard errors) of the differential intercept coefficients adjusted for other explanatory variables using multiple regression with nominal variables. Daughters of long-lived fathers (81+) are excluded from the analysis

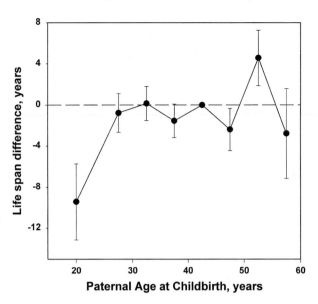

Fig. 6. Effect of paternal age at childbirth on daughters' life span based on 831 daughters from European aristocratic families born from 1800–1880. Daughters of longer-lived fathers (81+). Life expectancy of adult women (30+) as a function of father's age when these women were born (expressed as a difference from the reference level for those born to fathers aged 40–44 years). The data are point estimates (with standard errors) of the differential intercept coefficients adjusted for other explanatory variables using multiple regression with nominal variables

The data presented in Figure 5 are for daughters born to shorter-lived fathers (life span below 81 years). It is tempting to analyze the data for longer-lived fathers and to see whether the devastating effects of late reproduction will disappear. The rationale for such a prediction is based on the idea that mutations rates in both germ and soma cells depend on many common factors, including life style (exposure to carcinogens due to smoking, alcohol abuse, etc.) and genetic

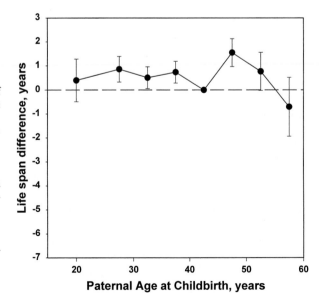

Fig. 7. Effect of paternal age at childbirth on sons' life span based on 10,103 sons from European aristocratic families born from 1800–1880. Life expectancy of adult men (30+) as a function of father's age when these men were born (expressed as a difference from the reference level for those born to fathers of 40–44 years). The data are point estimates (with standard errors) of the differential intercept coefficients adjusted for other explanatory variables using multiple regression with nominal variables. Sons of long-lived fathers (81+) are excluded from the analysis

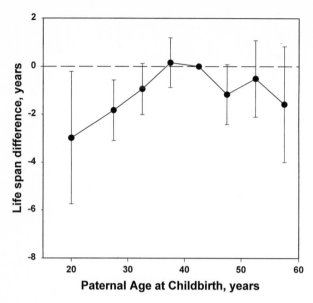

Fig. 8. Effect of paternal age at childbirth on sons' life span based on 1,912 sons from European aristocratic families born from 1800–1880. Sons of longer-lived fathers (81+). Life expectancy of adult men (30+) as a function of father's age when these men were born (expressed as a difference from the reference level for those born to fathers aged 40–44 years). The data are point estimates (with standard errors) of the differential intercept coefficients adjusted for other explanatory variables using multiple regression with nominal variables

predisposition. It is known that deficiency of vitamins B_{12}, folic acid, B_6, niacin, C, or E, appears to mimic radiation in damaging DNA by causing single- and double-strand breaks, oxidative lesions, or both, and may contribute to premature aging (Ames 1998). Therefore, those fathers who are fortunate for some reason to have low mutation rates are expected to live longer lives (because of less damage to their somatic cells) and also to produce healthy offspring with a normal life span in later life (because of less damage to their germ cells).

The results of data analysis for longer-lived fathers (81+) support the prediction that their progeny have normal life spans, even if conceived in old age (see Fig. 6).

Data for sons (Figs. 7, 8) demonstrate that a son's life span is not affected significantly by late conception, either by shorter-lived fathers (Fig. 7) or by longer-lived fathers (Fig. 8). This observation supports the previous finding that the life-shortening effect of late reproduction on offspring life span is in fact sex-specific (only daughters are affected). Possible explanations for this sex-specific phenomenon were discussed earlier.

As for maternal age effects on offspring life span, they are negligible for sons (Fig. 9) and suggestive (slightly positive) for daughters (Fig. 10). These results are consistent with the previous findings obtained by analysis of contour life span maps (see earlier). Further studies on larger sample sizes are required to have enough life span data for those born to particularly old mothers (over 45 years).

One of the new intriguing findings of this study is the paradoxical observation that children born to particularly young fathers (under 25 years) live shorter lives. To explain this paradox we suggest a hypothesis that life span shortening is caused by the residual genomic imprinting of the germ cell DNA in particularly young males. Specifically, we hypothesize that the DNA of young males is hyper-

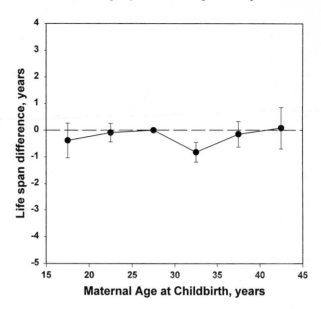

Fig. 9. Effect of maternal age at childbirth on sons' life span based on 12,015 sons from European aristocratic families born from 1800–1880. Life expectancy of adult men (30+) as a function of mother's age when these men were born (expressed as a difference from the reference level for those born to mothers aged 25–29 years). The data are point estimates (with standard errors) of the differential intercept coefficients adjusted for other explanatory variables using multiple regression with nominal variables

methylated and, for this reason, is more prone to mutations. Later in life, as males become more mature, their DNA is partially demethylated, so the risk of mutations may decline provisionally with age (25–30 years). After that time the mutation rate may start to increase again because of copy errors. It is known that the X chromosome is indeed methylated in the male germ line, whereas both X chromosomes are unmethylated in the female germ line (Driscoll and Migeon

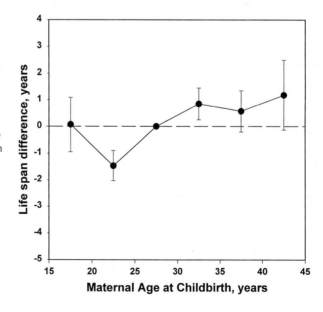

Fig. 10. Effect of maternal age at childbirth on daughters' life span based on 5,200 daughters from European aristocratic families born from 1800–1880. Life expectancy of adult women (30+) as a function of mother's age when these women were born (expressed as a difference from the reference level for those born to mothers aged 25–29 years). The data are point estimates (with standard errors) of the differential intercept coefficients adjusted for other explanatory variables using multiple regression with nominal variables

1990). This finding may explain why parental age effect on offspring life span is sex-specific: only paternal age is important, whereas maternal age effects are quite small, and also the affected sex is daughters only (who inherit paternal X chromosome). Further studies along these lines are required to allow us to test the proposed hypothesis as well as many other possible biological and social explanations. Collaboration in this area with other researchers and the IPSEN Foundation could shed light on the mechanisms of parental age effects that are of significant scientific and practical importance.

Acknowledgment

We would like to acknowledge support from the National Institute on Aging grants P20 AG12857, AG13698 and AG16138.

References

Abbott MH, Murphy EA, Bolling DR, Abbey H (1974) The familial component in longevity. A study of offspring of nonagenarians. II. Preliminary analysis of the completed study. Hopkins Med J 134:1–16

Ames BN (1998) Micronutrients prevent cancer and delay aging. Toxicol Lett 102–103:5–8

Aurox M (1983) La viellissement testiculaire et ses consequences. J Gynecol Obstet Biol Reprod (Paris), 12:11–17

Auroux M (1993a) Age du père et developpement. Contracept Fertil Sex 21:382–5

Auroux M (1993b) La qualité du conceptus en fonction de l'age du père. J Urol (Paris) 99:29–34

Auroux M, Mayaux MJ, Guihard-Moscato ML, Fromantin M, Barthe J, Schwartz D (1989) Paternal age and mental functions of progeny in man. Human Reprod 4: 794–797

Auroux M, Nawar NN, Naguib M, Baud M, Lapaquellerie N (1998) Post-pubescent to mature fathers: increase in progeny quality? Human Reprod 13: 55–59

Beeton M, Pearson K (1901) On the inheritance of the duration of life and the intensity of natural selection in man. Biometrika 1:50–89

Bertram L, Busch R, Spiegl M, Lautenschlager NT, Müller U, Kurz A (1998) Paternal age is a risk factor for Alzheimer disease in the absence of a major gene. Neurogenetics 1:277–280

Bocciolone L, Parazzini F, Fedele L, Acaia B, Candiani GB (1989) L'epidemiologia dell'aborto spontaneo: una revisione della letteratura. Ann Ostet Ginecol Med Perinat 110:323–34

Bocquet-Appel JP, Jakobi L (1991) La transmission familiale de la longévité à Arthez d'Asson (1685–1975). Population 46:327–47

Bordson BL, Leonardo VS (1991) The appropriate upper limit for semen donors: a review of the genetic effects of paternal age. Ferlil Steril 56:397–401

Bucher K, Ionasescu V, Hanson J (1980) Frequency of new mutants among boys with Duchenne muscular dystrophy. Am J Med Genet 7:27–34

Buffon J (1826) Oeuvres complètes de Buffon. Vol. 4 Paris, P. Duménil (Original edition 1749)

Carothers AD, Filippi G (1988) Klinefelter's syndrome in Sardinia and Scotland. Comparative studies of parental age and other aetiological factors in 47, XXY. Human Genet 81:71–5

Carothers AD, Collyer S, De Mey R, Frackiewicz A (1978) Parental age and birth order in the aethiology of some sex chromosome aneuploidies. Ann Human Genet 41:277–87

Carothers AD, McAllion SJ, Paterson CR (1986) Risk of dominant mutation in older fathers: evidence from osteogenesis imperfecta. J Med Genet 23: 227–30

Connor JM, Evans DA (1982) Genetic aspects of fibrodysplasia ossificans progressiva. J Med Genet 19:35–9

Crow JF (1993) How much do we know about spontaneous human mutation rates? Environ Mol Mutagen 21:122–29

Crow JF (1995) Spontaneous mutation as a risk factor. Exp Clin Immunogenet 12:121–28

Crow JF (1997) The high spontaneous mutation rate: Is it a health risk? Proc Natl Acad USA 94: 8380–86

Crow JF (1999) The odds of losing at genetic roulette. Nature 397(6717):293–4

Desjardins B, Charbonneau H (1990) L'héritabilité de la longévité. Population 45:603–15

Doblhammer G (1999) Longevity and month of birth: evidence from Austria and Denmark. Demograph Res [Online], vol. 1(3): 1–22. Available: http://www.demographic-research.org/Volumes/Vol1/3/default.htm

Driscoll DJ, Migeon BR (1990) Sex difference in methylation of single-copy genes in human meiotic germ-cells – implications for X-chromosome inactivation, parental imprinting, and origin of CpG mutations. Somat Cell Mol Genet 16:267–82

Erickson JD (1978) Down syndrome, paternal age, maternal age and birth order. Ann Human Genet 41:289–98

Eyre-Walker A, Keightley PD (1999) High genomic deleterious mutation rates in hominids. Nature 397(6717):344–7

Finch CE (1990) Longevity, senescence and the genome. Chicago, University of Chicago Press

Fretts RC, Schmittdiel J, McLean FH, Usher RH, Goldman MB (1995) Increased maternal age and the risk of fetal death. New Engl J Med 333:953–7

Friedman JM (1981) Genetic disease in the offspring of older fathers. Obstet Gynecol 57:745–9

Gavrilov LA, Gavrilova NS (1997a) Parental age at conception and offspring longevity. Rev Clin Gerontol 7:5–12

Gavrilov LA, Gavrilova NS (1997b) When fatherhood should stop? Science 277:17–18

Gavrilov LA, Gavrilova NS (1999a) How human longevity and species survival could be compatible with high mutation rates. J Anti-Aging Med 2(2):153–154

Gavrilov LA, Gavrilova NS (1999b) Season of birth and human longevity. J Anti-Aging Med 2(4):365–366

Gavrilov LA, Gavrilova NS, Snarskaya NP, Semenova VG, Evdokushkina GN, Gavrilova AL, Lapshin EV, Evdokushkina NN (1995a). Paternal age and the life span of descendants. Proc Russian Acad Sci [Doklady Akademii Nauk], 341:566–8. English translation published in Doklady Biological Sciences 341:196–8

Gavrilov LA, Gavrilova NS, Semyonova VG, Evdokushkina GN, Gavrilova AL, Evdokushkina NN, Lapshin EV (1995b) Human longevity genes are located in X-chromosome. In: Knook DL, Dittman-Kohli F, Duursma SA et al. (eds) Ageing in a changing Europe. III. European Congress of Gerontology: 30 August–1 September, 1995. Utrecht, Netherlands Institute of Gerontology, Abstract No 020.0027

Gavrilov LA, Gavrilova NS, Kroutko VN, Evdokushkina GN, Semyonova VG, Gavrilova AL, Lapshin EV, Evdokushkina NN, Kushnareva YuE (1997a) Mutation load and human longevity. Mutation Res 377:61–62

Gavrilov LA, Gavrilova NS, Semyonova VG, Evdokushkina GN, Kroutko VN, Gavrilova AL, Evdokushkina NN, Lapshin EV (1997b). Maternal age and offspring longevity. Proc Russian Acad Sci [Doklady Akademii Nauk] 354:569–572

Gavrilov LA, Gavrilova NS, Semyonova VG, Evdokushkina GN, Gavrilova AL, Evdokushkina NN, Kushnareva YuE, Andreyev AYu (1997c) Parental age at reproduction as a predictor of human longevity. In: 16th Congress of the IAG [International Association of Gerontology], August 19–23, 1997. Book of Abstracts. Adelaide, 461–462

Gavrilova NS, Gavrilov LA (1999) Data resources for biodemographic studies on familial clustering of human longevity. Demograph Res [Online], vol. 1(4):1–48 http://www.demographic-research.org/Volumes/Vol1/4/default.htm

Gavrilova NS, Semyonova VG, Gavrilov LA, Evdokushkina GN, Gavrilova AL, Lapshin EV, Evdokushkina NN (1995) Biomedical basis of sex differential in human life span. In: Knook DL, Dittman-Kohli F, Duursma SA et al. (eds) Ageing in a changing Europe. III. European Congress of Gerontology. 30 August–1 September, 1995. Utrecht, Netherlands Institute of Gerontology, Abstract No. 020.0028

Gavrilova NS, Gavrilov LA, Evdokushkina GN, Semyonova VG, Gavrilova AL, Evdokushkina NN, Kushnareva YuE, Kroutko VN, Andreyev AYu (1998) Evolution, mutations and human longevity: the study on European royal and noble families. Human Biol 70:799–804

Gourbin C, Wunsch G (1999) Paternal age and infant mortality. Genus LV (1–2):61–72

Hawkins MR, Murphy EA, Abbey H (1965) The familial component of longevity. A study of the offspring of nonagenarians. I. Methods and preliminary report. Bull Johns Hopkins Hosp 117:24–36

Hook EB (1986) Parental age and effects on chromosomal and specific locus mutations and on other genetic outcomes in offspring. In: Mastroianni L, Paulsen CA (eds) Aging, reproduction, and the climacteric. New York, Plenum, 117–46

Jalavisto E (1950) The influence of parental age on the expectation of life. Rev Med Liège 5:719–22

Kuliev AM, Modell B (1990) Problems in the control of genetic disorders. Biomed Sci 1:3–17

Lian ZH, Zack MM, Erickson JD (1986) Paternal age and the occurrence of birth defects. Am J Human Genet 39:648–60

Lurie IW (1994) Genetics of the Costello syndrome. Am J Med Genet 52:358–9

Martinez-Frias ML, Ramos-Arroyo MA, Salvador J (1988) Thanatophoric displasia: an autosomal dominant condition? Am J Med Genet 31:815–20

McIntosh GC, Olshan AF, Baird PA (1995) Paternal age and the risk of birth defects in offspring. Epidemiology 6:282–8

McVean GT, Hurst LD (1997) Evidence for a selectively favourable reduction in the mutation rate of the X chromosome. Nature 386:388–92

Meacham RB, Murray MJ (1994) Reproductive function in the aging male. Urol Clin North Amer 21:549–56

Miyata T, Kuma K, Iwabe N, Hayashida H, Yasunaga T (1990) Different rates of evolution in autosome-, X chromosome, and Y chromosome-linked genes: hypothesis of male-driven molecular evolution. In: Takahata N, Crow J (eds) Population biology of genes and molecules. Tokyo, Baifukan, 341–57

Murphy EA (1978) Genetics of longevity in man. In: Schneider EL (ed) The genetics of aging. New York, Plenum Press, 261–301

Olshan AF, Schnitzer PG, Baird PA (1994) Paternal age and the risk of congenital heart defects. Teratology 50:80–84

Orgel LE (1963) The maintenance of accuracy of protein synthesis and its relevance to aging. Proc Natl Acad Sci USA 49:512–17

Orgel LE (1970) The maintenance of the accuracy of protein synthesis and its relevance to ageing: A correction. Proc Natl Acad Sci USA 67:1476

Parazzini F, La Vecchia C, Mezzanotte G, Fedele L (1990) Maternal cohort, time of stillbirth, and maternal age effects in Italian stillbirth mortality. J Epidemiol Commun Health 44:152–54

Pearl R (1931) Studies on human longevity. IV. The inheritance of longevity. Preliminary report. Human Biol 3:245–69

Pearl R, Dewitt R (1934) Studies on human longevity. VI. The distribution and correlation of variation in the total immediate ancestral longevity of nonagerians and centenarians, in relation to the inheritance factor in duration of life. Human Biol 6:98–222

Perls TT, Alpert L, Fretts RC (1997) Middle-aged mothers live longer. Nature 389:133

Philippe P (1980) Longevity: some familial correlates. Soc Biol 27:211–19

Resseguie LJ (1976) Comparison of longitudinal and cross-sectional analysis: maternal age and stillbirth ratio. Am J Epidemiol 103:551–9

Risch N, Reich EW, Wishnick MM, McCarthy JG (1987) Spontaneous mutation and parental age in humans. Am J Human Genet 41:218–48

Robine J-M, Allard M (1997) Towards a genealogical epidemiology of longevity. In: Robine JM, Vaupel JW, Jeune B, Allard M (eds) Longevity: to the limits and beyond. Berlin, Heidelberg, Springer-Verlag, 121–29

Rogers JG, Chase GA (1979) Paternal age effect in fibrodysplasia ossificans progressiva. J Med Genet 16:147–8

Savitz DA, Schwingl PJ, Keels MA (1991) Influence of paternal age, smoking, and alcohol consumption on congenital anomalies. Teratology 44:429–40

Saxen L (1983) Twenty years of study of the etiology of congenital malformations in Finland. Issues Rev Teratol 1:73–110

Sheffield LJ, Danks DM, Mayne V, Hutchinson AL (1976) Chondrodysplasia punctata – 23 cases of a mild and relatively common variety. J Pediatr 89:916–23

US Bureau of the Census (1997) Statistical Abstract of the United States: 1997. 117th Edition. Washington DC

US Monthly Vital Statistics Report (1997) Volume 45, No. 11S, p. 44

Van Hueck W (ed) (1977–1997) Genealogisches Handbuch des Adels. Limburg an der Lahn, Germany, C.A. Starke Verlag

Vogel F (1983) Mutation in man. In: Emery AEH, Rimon D (eds) Principles and practices of medical genetics. London, Churchill Livingstone, 20–46

Vogel F, Motulsky AG (1997) Human genetics. Problems and approaches. Berlin, Springer-Verlag

Vijg J, Gossen JA (1993) Somatic mutations and cellular aging. Comp Biochem Physiol 104B:429–37

Wang TS, Pearson BE, Suomalainen HA, Mohandas T, Shapiro LJ, Schroder J, Korn D (1985) Assignment of the gene for human DNA polymerase alpha to the X chromosome. Proc Natl Acad Sci USA 82:5270–5274

Wyshak G (1978) Fertility and longevity of twins, sibs, and parents of twins. Soc Biol 25:315–330

Young ID, Thompson EM, Hall CM, Pembrey ME (1987) Osteogenesis imperfecta type IIA: evidence for dominant inheritance J Med Genet 24:386–9

Gender-Linked Effects on the Inheritance of Longevity
A Population-Based Study: Valserine Valley XVIII–XXth Centuries

A. Cournil

Introduction

The study of the inheritance of human longevity has long been of interest to scientists (Cohen 1964). Since one of the first studies done by (Beeton and Pearson 1901), many others have been accumulating empirical evidence pointing in the direction of a family component in the variability of life span (Pearl 1931; Jalavisto 1951; Abbott et al. 1974; Philippe 1978; Wyshak 1978; Bocquet-Appel and Jakobi 1990; Desjardins and Charbonneau 1990; Tallis and Leppard 1997; Cournil et al. 2000). This family component, also called the heritable component, is the product of the expression of shared characteristics between the members of a family. These characteristics can have two types of origin: genetic or environmental. The heritable component is generally assumed to correspond mainly to the genetic contribution (Falconer 1981) which might in some cases be a reasonable assumption in light of some careful studies conducted on twin population, where the heritability of life span is estimated to be about 20 to 30 % (Herskind et al. 1996; Iachine et al. 1998). Human population studies and other animal model approaches have led to a consensus among scientists regarding the existence of a low but consistent genetic component in the determinism of human longevity as well as of life span of other species (Curtsinger et al. 1995; Finch and Tanzi 1997).

The next step is to analyse whether we can "learn more" about this component and get some information about the underlying mechanisms of this inheritance. Many approaches have been developed to achieve this. For example, one strategy relies on the search for specific longevity genes, and has obtained encouraging results for several model organisms (Curtsinger et al. 1995). One of the best examples is *Caenorhabditis elegans*, a small worm nematode in which a single-gene mutation (age-1) leads to an increase in life span of 60 % (Friedman and Jonhson 1988). Emphasis has also been put on this kind of strategy for human populations since the beginning of the 90s through the so-called centenarians association studies. Several loci, like APOE or ACE, have been found to be associated with extreme longevity (Schächter et al. 1994). These kinds of studies are aimed at pointing out directly the fundamental, underlying genetic mechanisms that contribute to the determinism of longevity. Other more global approaches that are complementary to these approaches can be developed. In the case of human populations and family study, the goal is to estimate the heritabil-

Robine et al. (Eds.)
Sex and Longevity: Sexuality, Gender,
Reproduction, Parenthood
© Springer-Verlag Berlin Heidelberg 2000

ity of life span. A further step in these studies relies not on the analysis of the heritable component per se but on the factors that are susceptible to modifying the transmission of the character. The aim is to extract any specific pattern of variation of the heritability as a clue to get a better understanding of the underlying mechanisms and also to detect potential interactions between different processes. One example of this situation is suggested by the work of Gavrilov and Gavrilova (1997), who have detected a possible influence of paternal age at conception on daughters' life span. The father's age at conception would then be a typical factor that modulates the magnitude of the transmission.

Here, the main factor that we are going to focus on is the gender or sex factor. Sex is known to be an important determinant of survival and longevity (Gjonça et al. 1999). The sex-differential mortality has been extensively studied, and many theories and hypotheses covering the large spectrum from purely biological to purely environmental have been proposed to explain the difference (Smith and Warner 1989); but it is not yet completely understood. By contrast the influence of sex on the inheritance of life span has not been purposely investigated very often. The influence of sex generally refers to differences in heritability among males and females. For intergenerationnal approaches it can also refer to a differential influence of one parent's gender compared to the other (mother versus father influences). Some publications where the study design allows comparisons have mentioned some or no difference for the offspring or parental generation, but these results are generally found among a set of others results without providing any details or discussion. And the main problem arising from these observations is the strong heterogeneity of the results, which avoids any possible conclusions on this issue.

The main objective of this paper is to reanalyse the issue of gender effect on the inheritance of human longevity using a historical population register from a French rural region. Through the analysis of relationships between parents and children, we will address two distinct questions: 1) Is the heritability of longevity identical among sons and daughters? And 2) Is the influence of both parents on their offspring identical?

The other goal is a short review of previous family studies to analyse whether or not the heterogeneity of the results on the question of gender effect on inheritance can be explained. Before going further, it is important to clarify the conceptual framework of this study in regards to the definitions of longevity and heritable component. The definition of longevity varies from study to study (Wilmoth and Horiuchi 1999). It sometimes refers to the maximum life span of a species, or to the mean life expectancy of a population, or may also be used in the sense of a very long life, an exceptional length of life (Jeune and Vaupel 1995). Here, longevity refers to late or post-reproductive survival. Indeed, analyses are based on mean conditional life expectancy at a minimum age of 50 years for both generations, parents and children. This is an important and specific feature of our approach which distinguishes it from other family studies. Heritability is also a term that can have various definitions that sometimes lead to confusion (Jacquard 1983). Here, heritability is used as a measure of resemblance between parents and offspring. It can be considered as the additive genetic part contributing to the variation of the character (i.e. narrow sense heritability) conditionally to the assumption of no shared environment, which of course needs to be discussed (Kempthorne and Tandon 1953).

Valserine Population

Our data come from a data set that reconstructs the population of five adjacent villages located in a narrow valley of the French Jura mountains, near the Swiss frontier 10 km west of Geneva. This region is a rural area where about 90 % of the inhabitants are farmers, thus making the study population quite homogeneous with regard to socio-economic status and life style. The reconstruction of the population was carried out through the analysis of all parochial and civil registers available (Bideau et al. 1992). Data from approximately 70,000 vital events, such as births, marriages, and deaths from 1680 to 1980, have been recorded, making a file of about 46,000 individuals. From this data base, analyses were carried out from a sample of 643 nuclear families (parents and children) settled in the valley, in whom the parental dates of birth span a period from 1745 to 1849. Each member of the selected parental couples reached at least 50 years of age. The total sample contains 3,447 children; 2,389 of them, that had accurate dates of death were used in the analyses. We verified that missing data for the children were distributed homogeneously for sex and parental longevity.

Methodological Approach for the Estimation of Hereditary Effects

To estimate hereditary effects on longevity, we compared the mean life expectancies of offspring born of different kinds of parents who were categorized as being either "short-lived" or "long-lived". These two parental phenotypes were defined according to a selection of a percentile of the age-at-death distribution (Figure 1). For example, percentile 30 defines "long-lived" individuals as being those in the upper 30 % of the age-at-death distribution and "short-lived" individuals as being those belonging to the remaining fraction of the distribution. The selection was performed separately for six different distributions, for each sex and for three successive birth cohorts. Samples obtained from each cohort were then pooled for each phenotype and each sex. This pooling was done to avoid a selection bias stemming from an increase in life expectancy over time. The different combinations of the two phenotypes of both parents led to four types of parental couples (Figure 1): A, short-lived mother, short-lived father; B, long-lived mother, short-lived father; C, short-lived mother, long-lived father; D, long-lived mother, long-lived father.

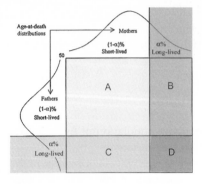

Fig. 1. Schematic description of the study design for the definition of the four parental groups. The percentile α refers to the upper fraction of the age-at-death distributions and defines the long-lived individuals

Pattern of inheritance

Global Hereditary Effects

Global hereditary effects were estimated on a sample of 1,102 children who had died after the age of 55. This sample contained 516 daughters and 586 sons with average longevities (above age 55) of 72.6 ± 0.4 and 72.3 ± 0.3, respectively. Thus, for this generation, no difference was observed between males and females with regard to mortality.

Effect of parental phenotype was estimated by comparing offspring having two long-lived parents (group D) to offspring having two short-lived parents (group A). Figure 2a shows the difference (D – A) for mean life expectancies at age 55 for the total sample of offspring and for different percentiles in a range of 20 to 35 %. The (D – A) differences appeared to be positive and statistically significant for all percentiles. The largest difference was observed at percentile 30, where offspring from group D (having two long-lived parents) lived on average 3.6 years longer than offspring from the group A (having two short-lived parents).

The effect of parental phenotype appeared to be rather stable for the different percentiles in a range of 20 to 35 %. This range corresponds to the definitions of parental longevity groups associated with the strongest influences on the offspring's longevity. Out of this optimal range the influence decreased.

Figure 2b presents the difference (D – A) for daughters and sons separately, and reveals a strong gender difference. The effect of parental phenotype proved to be stronger for daughters. The highest (D – A) difference is 6 years for daughters at percentile 20 whereas it is only 2.1 years for sons at percentile 25. Compared to daughters, hereditary effects on sons appeared to be very weak. This gap between males and females for the difference (D – A) was in fact essentially due to a difference in mean life expectancies for group D. For example, at percentile 20, the mean life span above 55 was 73.0 for males compared to 77.2 for females. However, no difference was observed between males and females for mean life spans of group A.

Both sons and daughters having short lived parents had lower mean life expectancies at age 55 than their counterparts having long lived parents. The dif-

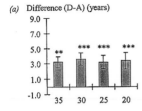

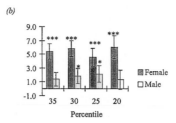

Fig. 2. Hereditary effects on offspring's longevity. Hereditary effects (*a*) for the total sample of off-spring an (*b*) for sons and daughters separately are represented by the differences (in years) and standard errors associated between life expectancies at age 55 of offspring in group D (two long-lived parents) and offspring in group A (two short-lived parents) for four different percentiles. p-values for t-test comparisons: * $p > 0.05$; ** $p < 10^{-2}$; *** $p < 10^{-3}$

ference was substantially larger for daughters compared to sons, thus indicating an effect of parental phenotype dependent on the offspring's gender.

Specific Parental Effects

Specific parental effects referred to separate estimates of maternal and paternal effects. They were estimated by the comparisons between offspring having a short lived father (belonging to the group A + B) to offspring having a long lived one (C + D) for the paternal effect and having a short lived mother (A + C) versus a long lived one (B + D) for the maternal effect. Figure 3 shows the differences (C + D) – (A + B) (father's effect) and (B + D) – (C + A) (mother's effect) of mean life spans above age 55 for each offspring's gender for the different percentiles. All the differences were found to be positive. For daughters, the paternal effect appeared to be stronger than the maternal effect at all percentiles. For sons, the predominance of one parent's effect over the other is less clear, but we can still observe a trend of stronger mother effects at percentiles 35 and 30. A way to test for the predominance of the influence of one parent over the other is to compare groups B and C. For daughters a predominant paternal effect would lead to a higher mean life expectancy in group C (long lived father and short lived mother) compared to group B (short lived father and long lived mother). A predominant mother's effect would lead to the reverse situation: B > C. None of the

Fig. 3. Specific parental effects on offspring's longevity. Specific parental effects are represented by the differences (in years) between life expectancies at age 55 of offspring. (C + D) – (A + B) for father/daugther and father/son. (B + D) – (A + C) for mother/daughter and mother/son

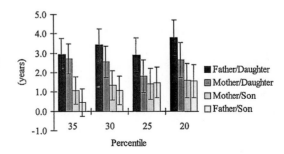

comparisons between groups B and C were statistically significant at a 5 % level. So, although a trend of a stronger paternal effect was observed for daughters, no definitive conclusions can be made concerning a gender linked differential parental effect, at least based on these preliminary analyses.

Age-Dependent Effect of Parental Phenotype

Before discussing these results, we have attempted to compare them with other studies on the transmission of longevity. First of all, it is important to point out that very few studies are completely comparable with ours. Indeed, some studies do not separate male and female offspring (Bocquet-Appel and Jakobi 1990) or only focus on one gender (Tallis and Leppard 1997), others do not separate specific parental effects (paternal and maternal) and finally almost none of them really tests (i.e. in a statistical way) for the existence of a gender effect. Their conclusions are based on observations. Despite all these difficulties, it remained possible to make partial comparisons with some studies. The major conclusion of the review is the great heterogeneity of results from the various studies. As a consequence, some results were contradictory to ours. For example, some authors reported a stronger maternal than paternal influence and a weak father-daughter correlation (Jalavisto 1951; Abbott et al. 1974; Philippe 1978). Other results were more consistent, like Wyshak (1978), who found a slight father's advantage, or identical paternal and maternal effect, and (Gavrilova et al. 1998), showing a stronger father-daughter correlation compared to father-son.

Faced with such a situation, we were prompted to ask whether some explanations could be found for this diversity. A detailed analysis of the studies suggested an important role of one criterion of the study design, which is the selection of the age-at-death groups. Indeed, reconsidering the above-cited example, it appeared that the former studies had taken infant or early adult mortality of the offspring into account, whereas the latter had been partially or completely restricted to mature adult mortality, as in our study. The choice of the age-at-death cut-off reflects in some way the definition taken into account for longevity, and appears to be very variable among the different works, often as a consequence of particular constraints of the data set. For example, taking into account younger ages allows bigger sample sizes. This situation has led us to test directly for the influence of the choice of this parameter on the pattern of inheritance. Here, we only focused on the offspring's age group. The parental sample remained unchanged and corresponded to ages at death above 50. Figure 4 shows global parental effect on offspring measured as before by the difference (D minus A). The differences were computed for the percentile 30 between mean life expectancies at different ages from 0 to age 65. As shown in Figure 4, the magnitude of the parental effect depends on age group selection, but more importantly, the pattern of variation differs for males and females and is almost opposite. Indeed, whereas the effect is minimal at birth for women and reaches a peak for life expectancy at age 50, it is maximal at birth for men and decreases thereafter, reaching a minimal level at age 55. So, this result agreed with the hypothesis that

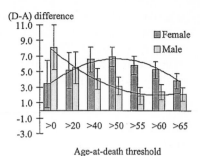

(D-A) difference

Fig. 4. Difference in conditional life expectancy at different ages in offspring from groups A and D. The differences (in years) (mean ± s.e.) between life expectancies of groups A and D are computed for different ages and for percentile 30

Age-at-death threshold

conclusions with regard to stronger hereditary effects for females or males depended on the study design. Studies taking into account young or young-adult ages-at-death will preferentially conclude that there is no difference or a weak stronger effect in males. One study of this kind is the Danish twin study (Herskind et al. 1996), where the authors have found heritability coefficients of 0.23 and 0.26 for females and males respectively, using a sample containing ages-at-death above 15 years. By contrast, studies focusing on later ages would preferentially conclude in favour of a stronger effect among females as we did. It is possible to go further by breaking up the global effect into specific parental effects. Figure 5a and 5b show paternal and maternal effects on each gender. As for global effect, the results indicate an influence of the age-at-death threshold in the pattern of inheritance, the influence being different between males and females. Comparison of maternal and paternal effects on one gender also reveals that the pattern of variation differs with regard to the gender of the parent. This is especially striking for females, where the pattern of variation with age of hereditary effects from father and mother is almost opposite. We observe here that the weak parental effect noted for females in Figure 4 when all ages were taken into account, was in fact due to a very weak father/daughter correlation, whereas

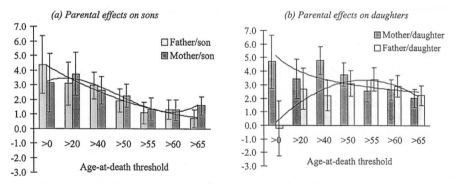

Fig. 5. Specific parental effects on offspring's life expectancy at different ages (*a*) for sons and (*b*) for daughters. Specific parental effects are represented by the differences (in years) between life expectancies of offspring for percentile 30. (C + D) – (A + B) for father/daughter and father/son. (B + D) – (A + C) for mother/daughter and mother/son

maternal effect is quite strong. This provides a clue to understanding why some studies have reported a stronger maternal effect and especially a weak father-daughter correlation. The age-group-related effect explains a consistent part of the contradictions found in the literature and also points out the importance of the study design in these approaches.

Discussion

The analysis of inheritance of longevity for our population of the French Jura has shown a consistent family component, as have many previous studies. Based on the characteristics of our population and study design, the family component observed is assumed to be mainly of genetic origin. The choice of a small, rural and homogeneous population and the sampling of the parental couples minimised environmental contributions in the family component. Restricting our analyses to post-reproductive survival in parents and children also reduced potential bias due to shared environment. An estimate of realised heritability [offspring's mean life span (D – A)/parent mean life span (D – A)] gave a coefficient of 0.27, which is in agreement with the heritability coefficients (0.26 for males and 0.23 for females) found in Herskind's twin study (Herskind et al. 1996). A heritable component is always population- and time-specific. In our case, we should point out that it is also age group-specific. Indeed, we have considered ages-at-death above 50 years for both generations. This particular feature of the study design enabled us to compare parents and children for the same range of variation of the character, which is not the case for most of the family studies on longevity, which usually compare parents and children in two different ranges of ages-at-death. The choice of this particular age group also had the advantage of considering distributions that approximated a normal curve. These two characteristics make the sample more suitable to estimate heritability, because for this estimate the trait is assumed to be quantitative.

As mentioned in the introduction, the goal of this work was to study the off-spring's and parents' gender-dependent effects in the inheritance of longevity. The analyses have clearly shown an influence on the offspring's gender. Indeed, the heritable component was found to be substantially larger for daughters compared to sons. No statistical evidence of differential influence of parental pheno-type according to the parent's gender was found. Still, a stable trend of a stronger effect of father's longevity compared to the mother's effect could be observed on daughters. Further analyses are necessary to confirm this trend. Finally, another important result came from the observation of age group-related effects on the magnitude and gender-related pattern of the heritable component. This latter result enabled us to explain a consistent part of the observed contradictions in the literature on the issue of gender effect in the inheritance of longevity.

The sex dependence of the heritable component of longevity might suggest cytoplasmic (mitochondrial DNA) or sex chromosomes-linked inheritance. Among the different hypotheses, the greater genetic variation for female offspring and the stronger father-daughter correlation suggested preferential X-linkage. The hypothesis of X-linkage for a longevity gene using an appropriate model is currently been tested on our population and appears to be fairly consistent.

The observed gender-linked pattern might also suggest different kinds of interaction between sex and genotype. Such interactions have already been observed in humans and in other species. For example, in a case-controlled genetic study of longevity, HLA-DR7 is associated with male centenarians only, whereas HLA-DR11 is associated with longevous women in long-lived sibships (Ivanova et al. 1998). In this regard, the recently reported linkage of type 1 diabetes to chromosome Xp in HLA-DR3-positive patients also provides direct evidence for an interaction between these loci in the aetiology of this autoimmune disease (Cucca et al. 1994). Interactions between genotype and sex are also found for Drosophila (Vieira et al. 2000). Finally, this interaction can also reflect an underlying environment × genotype interaction, if the contribution of environment in the variability of life span differs in male and female offspring (Herskind et al. 1996). We would then expect to find a greater impact of environmental factors for men. In view of our analyses, this hypothesis cannot be excluded even if no difference in survival was observed between males and females in our population, as normally observed for this region and time period.

These suggested explanations are only valid for the pattern observed for late survival, because our aim was to study determinism of late survival and to compare both generations for the same range of ages. However, it is clear that we have to take into account the variation of the pattern when considering younger ages, because late-age effects are probably not independent of what happened before as a result of selection processes.

This family study based on a well-defined population has revealed a particular gender-linked pattern in the inheritance of longevity and has suggested, among other hypotheses, a possible role of the X chromosome in the determinism of longevity. This work calls for replication in other populations to see whether the results and trends found in our population will find confirmation. Future work should also focus on alternative hypotheses that could explain the gender-dependent effects, especially through a model that takes into account the surprising result of the variation of the pattern with age.

Acknowledgements

We thank G. Brunet and A. Bideau of the "Centre d'Etudes Démographiques" for access to the data base and material support, and F. Schächter for his advice and help on this work. We are grateful to J-M. Robine and M. Allard for encouragement and support.

References

Abbott MH, Murphy EA, Bolling DR, Abbey H (1974) The familial component in longevity. A study of offsprings of nonagenarians. II. Preliminary analysis of the completed study. Hopkins Med J 134:1–16

Beeton M, Pearson K (1901) On the inheritance of the duration of life, and on the intensity of natural selection in man Biometrika. Vol. 1, pp 50–89

Bideau A, Brunet G, Heyer E, Plauchu H, Robert J-M (1992) An abnormal concentration of cases of Rendu-Osler disease in the Valserine valley of the French Jura: a genealogical and demographic study. Ann Human Biol 19:233–247

Bocquet-Appel J-P, Jakobi L (1990) Familial transmission of longevity. Ann Human Biol 17:81–95

Cohen BH (1964) Family patterns of mortality and life span. Rev Biol 39:130–181

Cournil A, Legay J-M, Schächter F (2000) Evidence of sex-linked effects on the inheritance of human longevity. A population based-study : Valserine Valley (French Jura), 18–20th centuries. Proceedings of the Royal Society of London. B 267:1021–1025

Cucca F, Goy JV, Kawaguchi Y, Esposito L, Merriman ME, Wilson AJ, Cordell HJ (1994) A male-female biais in type 1 diabetes and linkage to chromosome Xp in MHC HLA-DR3-positive patients. Nat Genet 6:29–32

Curtsinger JW, Fukui HH, Khazaeli AA, Kirscher A, Pletcher SD, Promislow DEL, Tatar M (1995) Genetic variation and aging. Annual Review of Genet 29:553–575

Desjardins B, Charbonneau H (1990) L'héritabilité de la longévité. Population 3:603–616

Falconer DS (1981) Introduction to quantitative genetics. Longman, London

Finch CE, Tanzi RE (1997) Genetics of aging. Science 278:407–411

Friedman DB, Jonhson TE (1988) A mutation in the age-1 gene in Caenorhabditis elegans lenghtens life span and reduces hermaphrodite fertility. Genetics 118:75–86

Gavrilov LA, Gavrilova NS (1997) Parental age at conception and offspring longevity. Rev Clin Gerontol 7:5–12

Gavrilova NS, Gavrilov LA, Evdokushkina GN, Semyonova VG, Gavrilova AL, Evdokushkina NN, Kush-nareva YE, et al. (1998) Evolution, mutations and human longevity: European royal and noble fami-lies. Human Biol 70:799–804

Gjonça A, Tomassini C, Vaupel JW (1999) Pourquoi les femmes survivent aux hommes? La Recherche 322:96–99

Herskind AM, McGue M, Holm NV, Sorensen TIA, Harvald B, Vaupel JW (1996) The heritability of human longevity: a population-based study of 2872 Danish twin pairs born 1870–1900. Human Genet 97:319–323

Iachine IA, Holm NV, Harris JR, Begun AZ, Iachina MK, Laitinen M, Kaprio J (1998) How heritable is individual susceptibility to death? The results of an analysis of survival data on Danish, Swedish and Finnish twins. Twin Res 1:196–205

Ivanova R, Henon N, Lepage V, Charron D, Vicaut E, Schächter F (1998) HLA-DR alleles display sex-dependent effects on survival and discriminate between individual and familial longevity. Human Mol Genet 7:187–194

Jacquard A (1983) Heritability: One word, three concepts. Biometrics 39:465–477

Jalavisto E (1951) Inheritance of longevity according to Finnish and Swedish genealogies. Ann Med Intern Fenn 40:263–274

Jeune B, Vaupel JW (1995) Exceptional longevity: from prehistory to the present Odense Monographs on Population Aging 2. Odense University Press, Odense

Kempthorne O, Tandon B (1953) The estimation of heritability by regression of offspring on parent. Biometrics :90–100

Pearl R (1931) Studies on human longevity. IV. The inheritance of longevity, preliminary report. Human Biol 3:245–269

Philippe P (1978) Familial correlations of longevity: An isolate-based study. Am J Med Genet 2:121–129

Schächter F, Faure-Delanef L, Guenot F, Rouger H, Froguel P, Lesueur-Ginot L, Cohen D (1994) Genetic associations with human longevity at the APOE and ACE loci. Nat Genet 6:29–32

Smith DWE, Warner HR (1989) Does genotypic sex have a direct effect on longevity? Exp Gerontol 24:277–288

Tallis GM, Leppard P (1997) Is length of life predictable? Human Biol 69:873–886

Vieira C, Pasyukova EG, Zeng ZB, Hackett JB, Lyman RF, Mackay TF (2000) Genotype-environment inter-action for quantitative trait loci affecting life span in Drosophila melanogaster. Genetics 154:213–227

Wilmoth JR, Horiuchi S (1999) Do the oldest-old grow old more slowly? In: Robine J-M, Forette B, Franceschi C, Allard M (eds) The paradoxes of longevity. Springer Verlag, Berlin, pp 35–60

Wyshak G (1978) Fertility and longevity in twins, sibs and parents of twins. Soc Biol 25:315–330

Genes and Centenarians

T. Perls, R. Fretts, M. Daly, S. Brewster, L. Kunkel and A. Puca

Nature Versus Nurture

It has been purported that aging was due to the interaction of many genes, perhaps eight to ten thousand, with weak effects interacting with one another and our internal and external environments. Yet genetic experiments in lower organisms and our own centenarian pedigree data indicate that at least a few genes may exist that exert a powerful influence upon longevity. Experiments in *C. elegans, Drosophila* and yeast show that the manipulation of one or a few different genes can result in the doubling to quintupling of life span. We have found that a sibling of a centenarian has a four to five times greater chance of reaching his/her early nineties compared to the sibling of someone who died his/her early 70s (Hitt 1999).

Additionally we have discovered several families highly clustered for extreme longevity. As will be discussed, the odds of encountering these families are fewer than one per all the families that exist in the world today, and thus they must have some shared advantage that allows them to exist. The patterns of inheritance that we are observing, in some cases Mendelian, make it extremely unlikely that a large number of specific allotypes could be simultaneously inherited to affect such a phenotype. Rather, it appears to us that a relatively few genes may have broad effects on how fast one ages and on susceptibility to diseases associated with aging.

In the nature versus nurture debate, those who claim that genes play a relatively minor role most frequently cite a highly popularized Danish study of monozygotic and dizygotic twins in which the heritability of life expectancy was noted to be about 25 % (McGue et al. 1993; Herskind et al. 1996; Finch and Tanzi 1997; Rowe and Kahn 1998). The problem is, however, that the oldest subjects in this study were in their mid to late 80s and the majority lived to average life expectancy (which in the United States is 76 years, about 74 years for men and 79 years for women). Differences in the environment accounted for 70 % of the variability in age at death for those with an average life expectancy. But these data do not tell us anything about the relative roles of genes and environment in the probability of achieving extreme old age. Thus it is safe to assume that average humans, born with an average set of genetic polymorphisms, will vary in their life expectancies according primarily to their habits and environments. But to live another 20 years, to age 100 and beyond, requires a distinct genetic advantage, the arguments for which we outline below.

Robine et al. (Eds.)
Sex and Longevity: Sexuality, Gender,
Reproduction, Parenthood
© Springer-Verlag Berlin Heidelberg 2000

Is living to 100 actually an advantage? If you believe that living the vast majority of your life in excellent health is a worthwhile goal, then the answer is yes. Centenarians probably achieve their extreme age by aging relatively slowly and either markedly delaying or in some cases escaping lethal diseases associated with aging. Nearly 90 % of centenarians in a New England population-based sample were functionally independent and healthy at age 92 and 76 % continued to be so at age 95. Even at an average age of 102 years, approximately 30 % were still doing very well. Centenarians reveal that the older you get, the healthier you've been rather than the long-held belief that the older you get the sicker you get (Perls 1995; Hitt et al. 1999).

Are Centenarians Genetically Different?

In 1825, Benjamin Gompertz proposed that mortality rate increased exponentially with age. Since then, most researchers have accepted that this rule indeed applies at younger adult ages for many species; however, at extreme old age, an exception to the rule exists. At very old age, mortality begins to decelerate in species such as medflies (Carey et al. 1992), *Caenorhabdititis elegans* (Brooks et al. 1994), and humans (Thatcher et al. 1996). Why does mortality decelerate? Most likely it is because frailer individuals drop out of the population, leaving behind a more robust cohort that continues to survive. Because these frail individuals drop out of the population, the distribution of certain genotypes and other survival-related attributes in a cohort changes with older and older ages. This selecting-out process is termed demographic selection.

The effect of demographic selection is exemplified by the drop out with extreme age of the apolipoprotein E ε-4 allele (Schächter et al. 1994). Rebeck and colleagues (1994) noted the frequency of the ε-4 allele to decrease markedly with advancing age. One of its counterparts, the ε-2 allele, becomes more frequent with advanced age. Presumably the drop out at earlier age of the ε-4 allele occurs because of its association with "premature" mortality secondary to Alzheimer's disease and heart disease. Recent investigation of the increased heritability of cognitive functional status at older age also supports the possibility that genetic polymorphisms may play an increasing role with older age (McClearn et al. 1997).

A similar trend exists in the case of the apolipoprotein B locus; where investigators from the Italian Centenarian Study comparing 143 centenarians with younger controls demonstrated an association between specific multiallelic polymorphisms and extreme longevity (DeBenedictis et al. 1997). In another study, nonagenarian subjects had an extremely low frequency of HLA-DRw9 and an increased frequency of DR1. A high frequency of DRw9 and a low frequency of DR1 are associated with autoimmune or immune-deficiency diseases that can cause premature mortality (Takata et al. 1997). Tanaka and colleagues (1997) demonstrated single nucleotide substitutions in three mitochondrial genes that were present in the majority of a small centenarian sample but rare in the general population. This study requires verification in other populations, given its small and homogeneous sample. Franceschi and colleagues (personal communications), when analyzing mitochondrial DNA haplogroups from 212 healthy centenarians and 275 younger controls, found that in male centenarians from Northern Italy, the J haplogroup was 10 times more frequent than in controls (23 % vs. 2 %; $p = 0.005$).

Such findings suggest that centenarians are ideal subjects for the discovery of other polymorphisms (or lack of polymorphisms) associated with a survival advantage. Furthermore, the apolipoprotein E ε-4 allele serves as an example of a polymorphism with an influence powerful enough to have a noticeable effect upon survival in the general population and across various ethnic lines. Wachter recently addressed the question of how many other such polymorphisms might exist. He argued, based upon the significant differences in mortality risk between people in their 90s versus those aged greater than 105, "there could be a relatively small number of genes – hundreds, not tens of thousands – which one has to not have in order to survive ad extrema." Of course, having the right polymorphisms may be as important as lacking the wrong ones (Wachter 1997).

Siblings of Centenarians Live Longer

In the course of recruiting centenarians in our population-based study, we frequently encountered subjects who reported similarly long-lived siblings. We therefore suspected that these siblings had genetic and environmental factors in common that conferred a survival advantage. To further investigate the question of familiality of longevity, we compared the longevity of siblings of 102 centenarians and siblings of a control group (n = 77) who were from a similar birth cohort born in 1896 but who died 27 years earlier at the age of 73 (Perls et al. 1998). The siblings of the centenarians had a substantially greater chance of surviving to extreme old age compared to the siblings of the controls. This relative risk of survival steadily increased with age for siblings of the centenarians, to the point that they had four times the probability of surviving to age 91 (Fig. 1). The relative risk for survival to older age continued to rise beyond age 91, though these larger differences were not statistically significant because of small numbers of siblings at these extreme ages. The observed trend was a 10 times greater risk of achieving age 95 and a 15 times greater risk of achieving age 100. These findings indicate that there is a strong familial component to extreme longevity but they do not distinguish between the relative importance of shared environmental and genetic factors.

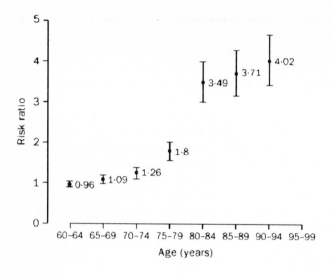

Fig. 1. Risk ratio of survival for siblings of centenarians versus siblings of 73-year-olds

Parents of Centenarians also Achieve Unusually Old Age

For 106 centenarians in our population-based sample, the mean age of their mothers was 75.5 years (n = 84, SD ± 18.6 years) and for fathers it was 74.4 years (n = 80, SD ± 16.6 years). These averages are higher than the average life expectancy of the time, which for Massachusetts residents, born in 1878-1882 who survived beyond the age of 20 years was 62 years for males and 63 years for females. A substantial proportion of parents achieved extreme old age; 21.6 % of mothers and 13.5 % of fathers survived to age ≥ 90 years.

Four Families with Clustering for Extreme Longevity

In gathering pairs of siblings as part of our Centenarian Study, we identified four families that clearly demonstrate segregation for extreme old age. We set out to expand these pedigrees and to determine if the clustering could be attributed to chance or if genetics must be playing a causative role. The pedigrees demonstrating vertical transmission of extreme longevity are shown in Figure 2.

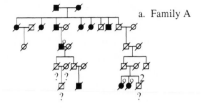

a. Family A

b. Family B

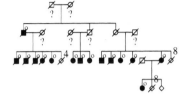

c. Family C

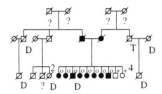

d. Family D

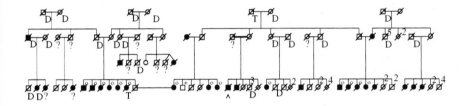

● ■ = age 90+ years

O = age verified
+ = age 80-89 years in good health
n = number of individuals
D = cause of death unknown
T = accident-related cause of death
? = birth and/or death date unknown
^ = discrepant data. age may be < 90

Fig. 2. Four families demonstrating vertical transmission of extreme longevity. Omitted family members died at age 18 years or younger or died at an age less than 90 years because of accidental trauma. The illustrated gender of certain members was altered for anonymity. Ages were validated using vital records and US federal census entries. *a)* Family A is composed of one male and four females aged 100 or older in one generation living in the 17th and 18th centuries. *b)* In family B, the individuals of note were born in the 19th century or early 20th century and seven are centenarians. *c)* In family C, there is a sibship of 13 children with eight reaching extreme old age (range: 90 to 102 years old). *d)* In family D, there are two branches linked together by marriage in the third generation. These different branches originate from the same small region in Norway. In the third generation, 23 of 46 individuals achieved extreme old age (range: 90 to 106 years old)

Mathematical Analysis

Cohort life tables for the years 1900, 1850 and 1801 were used to estimate the probability of individuals in Figure 3 surviving to their specified ages. For earlier birth cohorts, such as those encountered in the family A pedigree, the 1801 cohort life table was used as a conservative estimate of probability. These specific probabilities were then used to calculate a binomial probability of obtaining N individuals achieving their specified ages from a random sample of M individuals belonging to specific birth cohorts.

Probabilities were calculated for the single most impressive generation of each family. Probabilities would be even lower if the individuals achieving extreme old age from other generations were also taken into account.

The random chance of encountering the six siblings age 90 and older in family A is one in 10^9. In family B, there are three sibships that compose all grandchildren of two individuals. The chance of 13 of the 20 grandchildren living past 90 is about one in 10^{18}. In one of the three sibships, 5 of 16 siblings achieved age 100 or older, also an extremely rare encounter if left to chance. In the case of family C, the chance of eight siblings reaching at least 90 years is less than one in 10^{13}. Dominant inheritance is a possibility in this pedigree, given that both parents are affected and the children are largely or entirely affected. Though pedigree D appears to represent three unrelated branches, these branches originate from the same small region of Norway and therefore there may be a common ancestor. Nonetheless, treating the branches separately, the chance of encountering the 9 of 14 grandchildren reaching at least age 90 in the left branch is one in 10^{12}. The middle branch's grandparents had 12 of 38 grandchildren live to at least age 90,

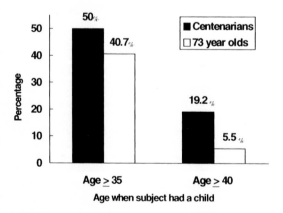

Fig. 3. Frequency of centenarian women and women surviving to age 73 years who gave birth at age 35 or older and at age 40 or older. Fifty percent of the centenarians had children at age 35 years or older compared to 40.7 % of the 73-year-olds. This difference was not statistically significant (odds ratio = 1.5, 95 % CI: 0.7–3.1, $P = .3$). 19.2 % of the centenarians had children at age 40 years or older compared to 5.5 % of the women who lived to age 73 (odds ratio = 4.0, 95 %CI: 1.02–18.7, statistically significant: $P = .02$)

a chance occurrence of one in 10^{11}. The right branch's grandparents had 8 of 26 also living to at least age 90; a chance observation of one in 10^8.

On the other hand, these probabilities would be higher if one were to take into account that these individuals, by virtue of having the same parents, had certain environmental characteristics in common that probably enhanced their ability to live beyond early childhood when there was a relatively high mortality risk. Such characteristics might include diet, hygiene, nurturing, socioeconomic status and so on. Reviewing the earliest life tables used in this analysis, we can conservatively reduce the above probability estimates by a factor of one hundred.

Even so, the above probability values remain smaller than one per the number-of-families-in-the-world today, so clearly there is familial aggregation that cannot be explained by random chance. Several points argue in favor of shared genetic factors, rather than environmental factors, effecting such a survival advantage. Two of the four families include cousins achieving extreme old age and these relatives are unlikely to have a common childhood environment. Also, the four described families come from distinct backgrounds. While this implies genetic as well as environmental diversity, one really cannot imagine any environmental components shared by these families that would be responsible for extreme longevity. Importantly, one would not necessarily expect that the families had the same genetic cause, but only that genetics plays an important role.

Middle Aged Mothers Live Longer: an Evolutionary Link Between Reproductive Success and Longevity-enabling Genes

As we reviewed the pedigrees of a number of our centenarian subjects living in the suburban Boston area, we came across a substantial number of women who had children in their 40s. There was even one that had a child at the age of 53 years. This struck us as unusual, given that maternal age greater than 40 is a relatively rare event. Less than 3 % of births occur in women 40 years of age or older (Fretts et al. 1995). In 1995 the birth rate of American women 40-44 years was 6.6 per 1000 women, and 0.3/1000 for women 45-49 (Ventura et al. 1997). However, a history of older maternal age among our centenarian subjects made sense to us since aging relatively slowly is a likely necessary characteristic of achieving extreme age, and women who do so should be able to bear children at an older age.

We went on to compare 78 female centenarians with a similar birth cohort of 54 women born in 1896, but who died at the age of 73 years in 1969. By collecting data on a similar birth cohort, we were able to minimize concerns about temporally related influences upon fertility such as health and contraception-related trends. We found that 19.2 % of the centenarians had children at age 40 years or older compared to 5.5 % of the women who lived to age 73 (Fig. 3). We concluded that, if you are a woman who naturally had a child in her 40s, you are four times more likely to live to be 100 years old than to die at the age of 73 (Perls et al.

1997). However, we believe that it is not the act of having a child in your 40s that promotes long life, but rather it is an indicator that the woman's reproductive system is aging slowly. A slow rate of aging would therefore bode well for the woman's subsequent ability to achieve very old age.

What are the factors that link the slowly aging reproductive system and the ability to reach extreme age? Ideally, to identify the reproductive factors that are associated with longevity we would like to know the status of various reproductive factors, such as age at menarche, cycle regularity, number of spontaneous abortions, and age of menopause. Unfortunately, obtaining this type of information from relatives of the deceased is difficult and unreliable. During the first quarter of this century, fertility-enhancing interventions for older women were not available. Under these circumstances, knowing when a woman last had a child is our best estimate of her premenopausal status and therefore reflects her natural ability to conceive later in life. Relatively delayed menopause, like pregnancy after age 40, may be a marker for aging slowly and the subsequent ability to achieve extreme longevity. This finding is interesting not only for its potential value in predicting individuals predisposed to extreme longevity, but also because it has implications regarding the theoretical basis of menopause and human life span.

The age of menopause was noted to be linked to longevity by Snowden et al. (1989), who studied 5287 white female Seventh-Day Adventists. The women who experienced menopause prior to the age of 40 had nearly twice the risk of dying during the study period compared to women who had experienced natural menopause at ages 50–54. This was true even after correcting for smoking, weight, reproductive history, and estrogen replacement. Because a history of estrogen replacement did not change these findings, it is possible that prolonged endogenous estrogen exposure is not the only explanation for the increased longevity of women with relatively delayed menopause.

In another chapter appearing in this monograph, Lund and Kumle describe their studies of the relationship between childbearing patterns and longevity among Norwegian women. The authors accessed census data concerning more than 900,000 married women of whom, on follow-up, approximately 171,000 had died. Women who had their last child at or after the age of 35 demonstrated an 11 % reduction in mortality risk relative to those who had their last child prior to age 25 and a 4 % risk reduction compared to those having their last child between the ages of 25 and 34. Twenty-eight percent of women surviving to age 90 or older had six or more children compared to 4 % of women surviving to age 40.

The ability to have a child later in life is associated with extreme longevity. Prolonging the period of time during which a woman can bear children would allow them to have more of them and therefore they would be genetically more fit and more likely to pass their genes down to subsequent generations. We propose that an evolutionary driving force behind the development of longevity-enabling genes would be the pressure to prolong the period of time (age) that a woman can bear children and therefore have more of them. But just as there is an optimal age for menopause (see below), there is also probably an optimal number of children, where too many would decrease the chance of their survival and too few would lessen the evolutionary advantage relative to those parents with more children. Slowing down aging and delaying the onset of diseases associated with aging would also enhance the chances of a woman to care for her children until they could fend for themselves and obtain reproductive age. A case could be made, realizing how long women live beyond the age of menopause, that such genes could ensure their roles as effective grandparents in facilitating the survival of their grandchildren.

Thus, longevity-enabling genes may be closely linked to reproductive health; perhaps they effect it directly. It may also be that the evolutionary pressure to delay a woman's menopause for as long as possible is an important driving force behind defining the life span of humans.

Thomas Kirkwood proposed that a tradeoff in metabolic resources occurs between reproduction and somatic maintenance. The disposable soma theory, which he elaborates upon in another chapter in this monograph, intrinsically predicts a tradeoff between fertility and longevity. In a study of British aristocratic families, Kirkwood and Westendorp noted a decrease in fertility (the number of children) among those men and women achieving the oldest ages. These findings are not incompatible with our findings that middle-aged mothers live longer. In fact, the disposable soma theory predicts centenarians would have a history of delayed menopause since better longevity-enabling genes would allow the tradeoff between somatic and reproductive maintenance to occur later in life (Kirkwood, personal correspondence). Thus, centenarians with their delayed menopause would demonstrate greater fertility, not less. The oldest women in the aristocracy study had a mean age of 68 years (95 % CI: 65.7–70.4 years) and subjects achieving extreme old age did not exist in large enough numbers to be analyzed.

Thus, when humans were evolving, average life expectancy may have been such that the tradeoff between somatic and reproductive maintenance occurred at a significantly younger age. A well-accepted tenant of evolutionary theory is that the extremes drive the evolution engine. Those relatively few extreme cases of advanced age, which were associated with enhanced fertility, may have been the fuel behind the engine to developing longevity-enabling genes. So, is the evolutionary reason for longevity-enabling genes the selective pressure to extend the time during which women bear children, or is it the need to enhance the provision of metabolic resources to somatic tissues so that the tradeoff in resources between the soma and reproductive system occurs later in life? In fact, both forces could be at work and they probably overlap, resulting in extreme longevity as a complex genetic trait rather than a single, monogenic one.

Many of the genes affecting reproductive health are found on the X chromosome. For example, deletions of important genetic information found on this chromosome have been associated with various degrees of premature ovarian failure and have been identified in mother-daughter pairs (Veneman et al. 1991; Tharapel et al. 1993). Perhaps the X chromosome is the first place we should look for longevity-enabling genes. It is interesting to note that one reason why women may live longer than men is because they have two X chromosomes whereas men have one. In each cell, one of these two X chromosomes is randomly inactivated. It is possible that, with age, those cells with an X chromosome (and its specific genetic polymorphisms) that is relatively less conducive to survival will be weeded out. Meanwhile, cells with the more advantageous X will become relatively more prevalent with older age. A man, on the other hand, would essentially be stuck with the one X chromosome without any alternative to enhance the probability of survival.

What Determines When a Woman Will Go Through Menopause?

Given available records, we know in Western societies the median age of menopause has remained relatively constant over at least the past 100 years and occurs, on average, at about age 51 (Napier 1987). In contrast to this stability, the age of menarche has declined significantly as health and nutrition have improved. Swinging in the other direction, it is possible that unprecedented rates of childhood obesity are contributing to even earlier menarche (Herman-Giddens et al. 1997). The age of menopause is influenced by both environmental and inherited factors. Smoking, the most common environmental toxin to ovarian function, causes earlier menopause (McKinlay et al. 1985). Chemotherapy, radiation, and surgery are less common causes of premature ovarian failure. In terms of inheritance, the influence of genetic factors is just becoming elucidated. A recent study of mothers and daughters found that the age of menopause in the mother was a significant predictor of the age of menopause in her daughters (Torgerson et al. 1997). This is particularly true of early menopause. Again, we maintain that the genes that regulate when a woman goes through menopause may be closely linked to genes that regulate how fast we age, our life expectancy and life span.

Menopause: an Adaptive Response

Menopause may act evolutionarily as a sentry to protect the aging woman from the hazards of childbirth. We support Doris and George Williams' theory, developed in 1956, that as humans evolved and became able to achieve older and older ages, there came a point when survival during childbirth began to decline as a function of further aging and increased frailty (Williams and Williams 1957). Females who by virtue of some genetic mutations became infertile prior to the age of marked mortality risk had a survival advantage over those females who did not have this series of mutations. An equally important advantage of continued survival would be that the mother could continue to raise and assure the survival of her children beyond puberty as well as to assist in the care of her children's children. From an energy allocation point of view, there probably comes a point with older age when it becomes more efficient to care for the children one already has and to perform other work in the society than to devote that energy to pregnancy, childbirth, and breast feeding. In primitive hunter-gatherer societies, postreproductive women perform a large portion of the work. Therefore, menopause provides a survival advantage and a means of better assuring the passing down of one's genes to subsequent generations. Williams and Williams thus called menopause an "adaptive response" to the increased mortality risk associated with childbirth.

Why Menopause Does Not Occur in Other Mammals?

In other mammals, giving birth is literally more straightforward and any associated mortality risk is relatively low even at advanced age. In humans, on the other hand, the birth canal has several twists and turns that developed coincidentally with the evolution of erect posture. It is this tortuous and cumbersome birth canal in humans that causes much of the mortality risk associated with childbirth. Because there is relatively little mortality risk associated with bearing young in other mammals, there is no selective advantage for the development of infertility (menopause) to assure the mother's survival and the survival of the young she has already produced.

The pilot whale, which also spends a significant proportion of time in a postreproductive state, is one exception to the rule (Austad 1994). This example of convergent evolution (when two unrelated species have a similar characteristic) may be due to chance; however, it is interesting that the pilot whale also spends a significant amount of energy rearing its young. The mother pilot whale will suckle its young for up to 14 years after birth. Menopause may make sense in this setting, where raising the young requires a significant period of time and energy before they are independent of their parent.

Nonhuman Data Supporting the Association Between Delayed Reproductive Senescence and Increased Longevity

Our observation in humans that fecundity at older age is associated with longer life expectancy correlates with those made by Michael Rose in his selection experiments of fruit flies, in which the ability to produce eggs later in life also correlates with greater life expectancy (Hutchinson and Rose 1991). Working with millions of flies, Dr. Rose and his colleagues selected out and bred flies that were born from eggs laid by the oldest females. With each subsequent generation, this selection process yielded older and older flies and the life span was increased.

The "Menopause and Grandmotherhood As Adaptive" Debate

Not all evolutionary biologists agree that menopause evolved because it provided a selective advantage. Since average life expectancy has increased considerably within the last 100 years, some believe that menopause is a relatively recent phenomenon. These biologists assert that humans have "outlived" their ovaries and thus menopause is simply an artifact of an unexpected recent increase in life span beyond reproductive age. Firstly, though average life expectancy has increased markedly in just the past century, the human life span has been significantly longer than the age of menopause, probably since the time menopause evolved. There is no evidence to indicate that we have done something special as a species in even the past millennium that would facilitate a doubling or tripling of the human life span. Certainly there is evidence from Ancient Greece indicating elder statesmen living well into their 80s and early 90s. Secondly, if menopause was simply an artifact, we would not expect, over the course of evolution, a natural selection for genes that influence when menopause occurs. Contrary to this supposition, genetics does appear to play a role in when menopause occurs; and finally, the nonadaptive hypothesis begs the question of why the reproductive system would fail long before other systems, such as the cardiovascular system.

Craig Packer, also a contributor to this monograph, maintains that menopause is nonadaptive, based upon his studies of African lions and savanna baboons (Packer et al. 1988). However, "menopause" and grandmotherhood in these mammals have little to do with such phenomena in humans. For example, Packer indicates that no female baboon survived beyond age 27 and maternity is usually noted until age 21. Of 508 females surviving beyond age 10 years, 86 % had died by age 21. Thus for the vast majority of baboons, death occurs at or before the age at which "menopause" is observed. The oldest lion survived to age 17 and maternity was usually noted until age 14. Of the 1661 lionesses surviving past the age of 6 years, 88 % died before age 14. Again, the vast majority of females in that group died at or before the age female "menopause" was observed among the pride. These observations are obviously extremely different from what is observed among humans. Packer goes on to further assert that menopause "probably pre-dates any sort of advantage from grandmothering in our own species" (Packer 1999). Again little can be said from observations of lions and baboons about the relationship between menopause and the advantage of grandparenting in humans. The most striking and important difference between these species and humans is that female grandparents still bear young when their children are also bearing young. As a result nothing can be said about the potential evolutionary advantage of grandparenting in humans based upon Packer's data.

Ruth Mace, in her studies of Gambian demographic data, also described in this monograph, convincingly makes the case that maternal grandmothers are significant determinants of their grandchildren's survival (Mace 2000).

Alan Rogers, studying data from agrarian Taiwan collected in 1906, generated a mathematical model to estimate the genetic contribution of women with and without menopause (Rogers 1993). He estimated that more than one of 10 women would have to die from childbirth for there to be a net decrease in a woman's genetic contribution to subsequent generations. If maternal mortality was less than 10 %, he supposed that menopause would not be particularly adaptive. However, Rogers did not estimate and include in his mathematical model a variable that would sufficiently reflect the maternal energy that is required to ensure survival for her offspring and her children's offspring. Any estimate of energy required to raise a child to independence is likely to be underestimated. We argue that if both maternal mortality and maternal energy are considered, the evolution of menopause would be adaptive and increase the success rate for genetic contribution to future generations.

Why Is the Human Life Span 122 Years and What Is the Evolutionary Advantage for Living to Such an Age?

Based upon our observations, the slower a woman ages, the longer period of time and greater opportunity she has to produce children and thus contribute her genes to the gene pool. Despite the fact that menopause must still occur, a continued slow rate of aging and perhaps also a decreased susceptibility to diseases associated with aging that can cause maternal mortality would therefore allow a woman to achieve extreme longevity. From a Darwinian point of view, we assert that there is no selective advantage for humans to have a life span of approximately 100 years. Rather, attaining such very old age is simply a by-product of the genetic forces that maximize the length of time during which women can bear children. Just because a woman goes through menopause does not mean that the genes that allowed her to age slowly and have a decreased predisposition to age-related diseases suddenly turn off; these genes continue to exert their influence, and thus enable her to achieve extremely old age. In other words, menopause may be the evolutionary fulcrum that determines human life span. Where does that leave men in the scheme of things? We would argue that the purpose of males in our species is simply to pass down genes to their female offspring that facilitate the woman to age as slowly as possible.

What If We Removed the Selective Force for Maximizing Life Span?

Due to the tremendous advances of 20th century obstetrics, the mortality risk for the mother during childbirth has markedly declined. With this decline in risk there is no longer the pressure to age slowly to maximize the period of time during which women have the opportunity to bear children. Therefore, it is unlikely that natural selection forces will promote further expansion of the human life span.

The close relationship between genes that regulate reproductive fitness in women and genes that regulate rates of aging and susceptibility to diseases associated with aging is intriguing. To date, there have been no specific genes identified that promote later menopause; presumably they exist and are responsible for prolonged ovarian function. These ovarian function-promoting genes may be closely associated with longevity-enabling genes or they may somehow be one and the same. Perhaps such genes will be identified as the result of linkage and positional cloning studies of centenarian sib-pairs and families with multiple centenarians.

The evaluation of known candidate genes for polymorphisms occurring at frequencies that differ between centenarians and ethnically matched controls is another important approach, as illustrated by the aforementioned work with apolipoprotein E and its major polymorphisms. Numerous researchers have their favorite candidate genes for investigating the modulators of aging and its associated diseases (Schächter 1998). Clearly, the discovery of candidate genes in lower organisms is crucial for the identification of genes to be studied in human cohorts such as centenarians. The explosion of findings currently occurring from these different approaches appears to indicate that we should have key answers to the molecular genetics of the aging puzzle in the very near future.

Acknowledgments

We are indebted to the following: The Alzheimer's Association Darrell and Jane Phillippi Faculty Scholar Award, the National Institute on Aging (AG-00294 and R0-3), the Institute for the Study of Aging, The Retirement and Research Foundation and The Paul Beeson Faculty Scholars in Aging Research Program.

References

Austad SN (1994) Menopause, an evolutionary perspective. Exp Gerontol 29:255–263
Brooks A, Lithgow GJ, Johnson TE (1994) Mortality rates in a genetically heterogeneous population of *Caenorhabditis elegans*. Science 263:668–671
Carey JR, Liedo P, Orzoco D, Vaupel JW (1992) Slowing of mortality rates at older ages in large medfly cohorts. Science 258:457–461
De Benedictis G, Falcone E, Rose G, Ruffolo R, Spadafora P, Baggio G, Bertolini S, Mari D, Mattace R, Monti D, Morellini M, Sansoni P, Franceschi C (1997) DNA multiallelic systems reveal gene/longevity associations not detected by diallelic systems. The APOB locus. Human Genet 99:312–318
Finch CE, Tanzi RE (1997) Genetics of aging. Science 278:407–411
Fretts RC, Schmittdiel J, McLean FH, Usher RH, Goldman MB (1995) Increased maternal age and the risk of fetal death. New Engl. J. Med. 333:953–957
Herman-Giddens ME, Slora EJ, Wasserman RC, Bourdony CJ, Bhapkar MV, Koch GG Hasemeier CM (1997) Secondary sexual characteristics and menses in young girls seen in office practice: a study from the Pediatric Research in Office Settings network Pediatrics 99:505–12
Herskind AM, McGue M, Holm NV, Sorensen TI, Harvald B, Vaupel JW (1996) The heritability of human longevity: a population-based study of 2872 Danish twin pairs born 1870–1900. Human Genet 97:319–323
Hitt R, Young-Xu Y, Perls T. (1999) Centenarians: The older you get, the healthier you've been. Lancet 354 (9179):652
Hutchinson EW, Rose MR (1991) Quantitative genetics of postponed aging in *Drosophila melanogaster*. I. Analysis of outbred populations. Genetics 127:719–727
Mace R (2000) Evolutionary ecology of human life history. Anim Behav, in press
McClearn GE, Johansson B, Berg S, Pedersen NL, Ahern F, Petrill SA, Plomin R (1997) Substantial genetic influence on cognitive abilities in twins 80 or more years old. Science 276:1560–3
McGue M, Vaupel JW, Holm N, Harvald B (1993) Longevity is moderately heritable in a sample of Danish twins born 1870–1880. J Gerontol Biol Sci 48:B237–B244
McKinlay SM, Bifano NL, McKinlay JB (1985) Smoking and age at menopause. Ann Intern Med 103:350–356

Napier ADL (1987) The menopause and its disorders. London, Scientific Press

Packer C (1999) Reproductive cessation: adaptation or senescence? Abstract appearing in Sex and Longevity, sexuality, gender, reproduction and parenthood. Foundation IPSEN, October 18, 1999

Packer C, Tatar M, Collins A. (1988) Reproductive cessation in female mammals. Nature 392:807–811

Perls TT (1995) The oldest old. Sci Am 272:70–75

Perls T, Alpert L, Fretts R (1997) Middle aged mothers live longer. Nature 389:133

Perls T, Wager C, Bubrick E, Vijg J, Kruglyak L (1998) Siblings of centenarians live longer. Lancet 351:1560

Rebeck GW, Perls TT, West HL, Sodhi P, Lipsitz LA, Hyman BT (1994) Reduced apolipoprotein epsilon 4 allele frequency in the oldest old. Alzheimer's patients and cognitively normal individuals. Neurology 44(8):1513–1516

Rogers AR (1993) Evol Ecol 7:406–420

Rowe JW, Kahn RL (1998) Successful aging. New York, Random House

Schächter F (1998) Causes, effects and constraints in the genetics of human longevity. Am J Human Genet 62:1008–1014

Schächter F, Faure-Delanef L, Guenot F, Rouger H, Froguel P, Lesueur-Ginot L, Cohen D (1994) Genetic associations with human longevity at the APOE and ACE loci. Nat Genet (1994) 6:29–32

Snowden DA, Kane RL, Beeson WL (1989) Is early natural menopause a biological marker of health and aging? Am J Pub Health 79:709–714

Takata H, Suzuki M, Ishii T, Sekiguchi S, Iri H (1997) Influence of major histocompatibility complex region genes on human longevity among Okinawan-Japanese centenarians and nonagenarians. Lancet 2:824–826

Tanaka M, Gong JS, Zhang J, Yoneda M, Yagi K (1997) Mitochondrial genotype associated with longevity. Lancet 351(9097):research letter

Tharapel AT, Anderson KP, Simpson J (1993) Deletion (X) (q26.2 → q28) in a proband and her mother: molecular characterization and phenotypic-karyotypic deductions. Am J Human Genet 52:463–471

Thatcher AR, Kannisto V, Vaupel JW, Yashin Al (1996) The force of mortality from age 80 to 120. Odense, Denmark, University Press

Torgerson DJ, Thomas RE, Reid DM (1997) Mothers and daughters menopausal age: is there a link? Eur J Obstet Gyn 74:63–66

Veneman TF, Beverstock GC, Exalto N, Mollevanger P (1991) Premature menopause because of an inherited deletion in the long arm of the X-chromosome. Fertil Steril 55:631–633

Ventura JS, Martin JA, Curtin SC (1997) Report of final natality statistics, 1995. Centers for Disease Control and Prevention/National Center for Health Statistics. Bethesda

Wachter KW (1997) Between Zeus and the salmon: Introduction. In: Wachter KW, Finch CE (eds) Between Zeus and the salmon. The biodemography of longevity. Washington, DC, National Academy Press

Williams GC, Williams DC (1957) Natural selection of individually harmful social adaptations among sibs with special reference to social insects. Evolution 11:32–39

Evolutionary Ecology
of the Human Female Life History

R. Mace

Summary

The human female life history is characterised by several unusual features compared to other apes, including large babies, late puberty and a rapid reproductive rate, followed by the menopause. In this review I examine human life history from an evolutionary ecological perspective.

The evidence for life history trade-offs between fertility and mortality in humans is reviewed. Patterns of growth, fertility and mortality across the life span are illustrated with data from a traditional Gambian population. The stages of the human life course are outlined, followed by a discussion of the evolution of menopause – the curtailing of female reproduction long before death. The evidence that this stage evolved because investment in children's future reproductive success is more important than continuing childbearing into old age is reviewed, along with data relating to the biological constraints that may be operating.

Human Evolutionary Ecology

Humans have big but relatively helpless babies, infant mortality is high, sibling rivalry is fierce and puberty is late. For women, childbearing is rapid and dangerous, parental effort is arduous and protracted, and post-reproductive life is long. Whilst many of these characteristics are common to the apes, many are exaggerated or unique in *Homo sapiens*.

Humans are so unusual in so many respects that it is hard to attribute some aspect of their behaviour or life history to some aspect of their ecology by comparison with other primates. An outstanding oddity is the size of our brain, which lies two to three standard deviations above the line predicting brain size from body size for primates (Pagel and Harvey 1989); it is plausible (although far from certain) that many of the other unusual features of human life history relate back to this. The consequences of a large brain are both behavioural and physiological. In this review I will concentrate primarily on those aspects of human life history that are most related to our social system, but our social system has had a powerful influence on the evolution of our physiology as well as our psychology.

Human behaviour is hugely influence by culture, which is itself a by-product of our intelligence. So integrated are behaviour and culture that I shall use the

Robine et al. (Eds.)
Sex and Longevity: Sexuality, Gender,
Reproduction, Parenthood
© Springer-Verlag Berlin Heidelberg 2000

two words almost synonymously. We can decide when to mate and have children, how much to feed them and how long to live with them. These are either individual decisions or behaviours followed because we want to follow some cultural norm; most such decisions are a combination of both of these features.

Amongst those studying the evolution of human behaviour, the emphasis differs as to which theoretical framework is most likely to help us understand why we do what we do. Evolutionary psychologists have taken a view that much of our behaviour can be understood as genetically adapted to an ancestral environment in which we existed as hunters and gatherers for the vast majority of our evolutionary history. This ancestral environment is often referred to as our environment of evolutionary adaptedness (EEA), generally proposed as a dry, African savannah. This model draws heavily an one of the first hunter-gatherer groups whose life history was ever studied: the !Kung San of southern Africa (Howell 1979). These mild, monogamous, musical people with carefully spaced children provide an appealing candidate for the typical, ancestral human social unit. But the legends of !Kung life are faltering. Their famous four-year birth intervals retreated to the more common 2.5–3 years when !Kung were treated for sexually transmitted diseases (Pennington 1992), as did those of all the other populations in northwestern Botswana. And in Cavalli-Sforza et al.'s (1994) examination of human population history, the !Kung are described as an unlikely candidate for an ancestral African group that might even have migrated into Africa from Asia. Subsequent studies of other hunter-gatherers have exposed what any behavioural ecologist might have suspected, which is that there no clear case for a typical human ecology. In a recent study of the Ache of Paraguay (currently the most thorough examinations of forager life history), Hill and Hurtado (1996) describe a group that, in many ways, is much more likely to characterise ancestral humanity. The Ache had far less exposure to non-foraging groups than the !Kung. Forest-dwellers, they lived in fierce isolation until 1972, when they were devastated by epidemics caught from missionaries. Those that survived had to retreat to reservations. Their story revealed a life of hardship, violence within and between social groups and rapid reproduction. Infanticide and geronticide were common, family groups were unstable and few individuals lived long enough to contribute much to the social unit in post-reproductive life. Constant warfare between groups, with populations sometimes decimated, sometimes expanding rapidly into new areas, could easily be the circumstances in which our life history evolved.

Some evolutionary psychologists (e.g., Symons 1979) have argued that the origin of agriculture, which fuelled population expansion, was so recent that evolution would not have had enough time to change our behaviour since then, and thus there is little point in studying the fitness consequences of any behaviour in societies other than hunter-gatherers. However, there is evidence for genetic adaptation in humans since the origin of agriculture; for example the ability to digest lactose as an adult has evolved as an adaptation to dairying in groups that have been keeping cattle for less than 10,000 years (Simoons 1978; Holden and Mace 1997). It can be argued, convincingly, that workloads, reproductive experience and many other aspects of life history did not change nearly as much in the transition between foraging and peasant farming as they have over the last 200 years with the demographic transition to small family size (Strassman and Dunbar 1999).

Given that we do not know what our ancestors did, we cannot compare ourselves very meaningfully with other primates, and as humans are generally not amenable to experimental manipulation, we are left with an examination of the ecological and social correlates of individual and cross-population variation in human life history. Thus the methods of behavioural and evolutionary ecology are likely to be important. For human beings, their cultural environment is as much a given as any other part of their environment, so the tools of behavioural ecology have to be applied in a framework in which the environment includes culture.

I shall illustrate many aspects of human life history with data collected between 1950 and 1975 from a west African village. This dataset is one of the most complete records of the demography of a natural, food-limited, human population from Africa. It was collected, in real time, as part of a long-term medical research project based in a Gambian village where the population was reliant on agriculture and suffering high mortality. I chose this population to illustrate an evolutionary ecological view of human life history, not because it has any claim to being ancestral but only because it is a well-documented, traditional population that is as likely to be characteristic of humanity as any other.

Trade-Offs in Life History

Figure 1(a–c) illustrates the essential features of the human life history: growth, mortality and fertility. A fundamental assumption of life history theory is that trade-offs exist between energy expended an growth and factors influencing mortality an the one hand and reproduction an the other (Williams 1957; Roff 1992; Stearns 1992). The costs of reproduction may be paid in terms of energy being diverted away from body repair and maintenance (Kirkwood and Rose 1991) and reducing investment in immunological competence. Evidence for trade-offs between reproductive effort and life span has been gathered from experimental manipulation in numerous animal species (reviewed in Roff 1992). An obvious problem with gathering such evidence from humans is that researchers have had to rely an phenotypic correlations or "natural experiments." Phenotypic correlations are problematic, because heterogeneity in a population can obscure true relationships between life history variables. For example, if individual women are reproducing up to their own capacity, then healthier women have larger families and potentially greater longevity, but if that additional reproduction shortens life span, then no correlation between family size and longevity will emerge. Notwithstanding these problems, immediate costs both in terms of maternal mortality risk and nutritional stress after reproduction have been shown in malnourished populations (Tracer 1991). Lund (1990) found that women in Norway with fewer than four children lived longer than those with more than four children. Westendorp and Kirkwood (1998) used historical data to show that faster childbearing in women of the English aristocracy was associated with a shorter life span among those reaching advanced ages. They also found that late reproduction was associated with longevity, a finding also shown by Perls et al. (1997), which they interpreted as evidence of a genetic trade-off

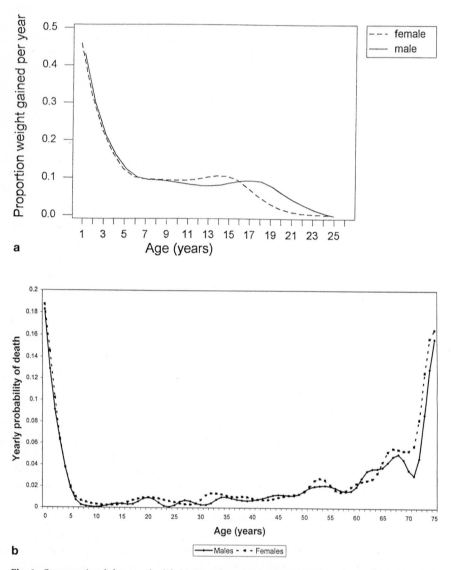

Fig. 1. Cross-sectional data on the life history of rural Gambians, based on data collected by Sir Ian McGregor from Keneba and Manduar villages between 1950 and 1975. *a)* Average annual weight gain as a proportion of total weight, between birth and 25 years of age for males and females. *b)* Annual mortality hazard for males and females over the life span.

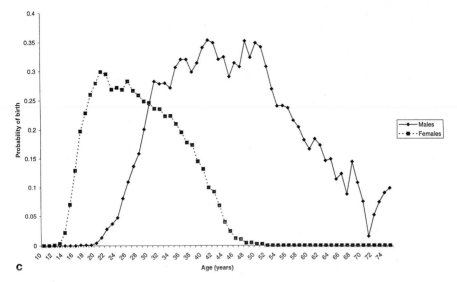

Fig. 1. *c)* Age-specific fertility (number of live births per year) for males and females over the life span (3 year running means)

between reproduction and longevity. It should be noted that these effects are rather subtle, and it is not clear that they are operating at biologically meaningful levels.

With respect to assessing the role of immune function in life history, most of the relevant research an humans has taken a different direction from that done an animals. This is due to the availability of data documenting variation in foetal nutrition, providing natural experiments which appear to show that gestation critical time for programming immune function in later life. Barker (1994) showed that poor nutrition in the womb, caused either by serious food shortages for mothers or medical complications during pregnancy, is associated with skinny babies and greatly increased risk of degenerative disease in late adulthood (such as diabetes and heart attack). Moore et al. (1997) used marked seasonality as a natural experiment to show that mothers in the third trimester of pregnancy in the hungry season in the Gambia had children that were more likely to die of infectious disease when they became adults. Whether diversion of energy away from the immune system in adult life mediates costs of reproduction has yet to be established.

Whatever the precise mechanisms of the costs of reproduction are, women around the world are certainly well aware of them. It is the optimal allocation of energy through the life course that is the challenge of human life history. Trade-offs are involved at every stage: trade-offs between growth and reproduction, between one child and another, between children and grandchildren. Life history theory is the only theoretical paradigm with the potential to predict how natural selection should resolve these trade-offs.

The Life Course

Birth and Infancy

Birth is difficult and painful in humans because of the large size of the baby and the fact that our upright posture necessitates a stiff pelvis. For most mammals brain growth slows at birth, but in humans, the skull is not fully hardened at birth to ease delivery and brain growth continues rapidly after birth for about one year, reaching adult size in about seven years (Bogin 1999).

Delivery is still risky for bath mother and baby. Maternal mortality varies enormously around the world, reaching a peak in hospitals with poor hygiene, where delivery can be more dangerous than at home. In countries with no effective modern medicine, the risk of death in childbirth outside hospital is less than 1 % per birth, but follows a j-shaped function, i.e., declines after the first birth, and then rises again in high parity women. The overall rate may be less than our fear of childbirth would lead us to expect, but, because adult mortality in humans is low, the less than 1 % risk of maternal mortality per birth typically translates into between 0.25 and 0.33 of all deaths of women of reproductive age in natural fertility populations (see Mace and Sear 1997 for African examples). Female mortality often exceeds that of males during their twenties and thirties for this reason. The provision of antibiotics and facilities for safe caesarian section and blood transfusion markedly reduces this risk (Graham 1991), and when these are available maternal mortality is negligible.

Risks for the baby are far higher. Except with the best medical care, perinatal mortality risk rarely falls below 1 %. Same of this mortality may be due to genetic defects which are only fatal after birth. In the Gambian example in Figure 1, the high end of the spectrum is illustrated: nearly 7 % of all infants born alive died within one month. Body weight is a strong and consistent correlate of an infant's chance of surviving its first year. Weaning is a hazardous time, as infants are exposed to less nutritious food and unclean water. The earlier children are weaned, the higher is infant mortality. The most common reason for weaning is a subsequent pregnancy; and the evidence that closely spaced birth greatly increases infant mortality is overwhelming (Hobcraft et al. 1983; Alam 1995; Bohler and Berghoff 1995). Older siblings then compete for food (LeGrand and Philips 1996).

Human babies are also at risk from infanticide or neglect leading to reduced survival. The classic scenario outlined for numerous mammals – infanticide by incoming males, so as to redirect a mother's parental effort towards the new males' future offspring – was shown to be a serious risk to children under two in our own society by Daly and Wilson (1985). Voland (1988) found statistical evidence from 18th century Germany that women who were widowed when young may have been depressing the survival chances of their young children to enhance their prospects of remarriage. Again, something similar appears in our own back yard (Daly and Wilson 1996). Abandonment of the mother by her husband is frequently associated with infanticide, often at birth (e.g., among the

Ache; Hill and Hurtado 1996). Sex preferences can also cause significant sex biases in infant and child mortality. These biases can be against girls (as often found in patrilineal societies, particularly in Asia) or against boys (particularly in matrilineal societies, such as in southern Africa; Harpending and Pennington 1991). Children of the least favoured sex who have older siblings of the same sex are at particular risk (DasGupta 1987). Most of these patterns which indicate parental influence in childhood mortality have been discerned by careful statistical analysis of demographic data rather than by interviews with parents. However, when economic conditions and levels of kin and paternal support are dreadful, mothers do sometimes admit to their unwilling compliance in infanticide by neglect, as Scheper-Hughes (1992) described in Brazilian shantytowns.

Faced with the hazards of babyhood, there is little the baby can do about it except grow up as fast as possible (Fig. 1a). As children grow, they require less intense parental effort, and as they escape into the oasis of childhood they appear to be less at risk of mortality in general (Fig. 1b).

Childhood and Puberty

Childhood is not unique to humans, with something similar being found in other apes (Perriera and Fairbanks 1991), but in humans it is especially prolonged. Childhood is generally assumed to be about intellectual and social, rather than physical, development (Bogin 1999), although there are same dissenters from this view (Burton-Jones et al. 1999). Hard evidence that what we learn in childhood contributes to our fitness is conspicuous by its absence. Catch-up growth, shown by children recovering from illness or a period of malnutrition, illustrates that a much faster growth rate than that shown is physiologically possible. But adult-sized, fully developed 5-year-olds are a scary thought, and it is doubtful that they would he particularly successful in the competition for resources or mates with 20-year-olds. Better that a period of learning, or simply waiting, is protected in a state of lower nutritional requirements, less threat to adults and low mortality. Along similar lines, Haig (1999) describes childhood as a strategy to extract more parental investment.

When children reach puberty, they spurt in growth to at or near their full height. This adolescent growth spurt is uniquely human. Figure 1a shows average weight gain for children of each age, but individual growth curves would show pronounced spurts, which are averaged out here. Growth spurts are more pronounced in well-nourished than in malnourished populations, such as in this Gambian case. Males achieve greater average adult height than females in all populations studied, although cross-population variation in sexual dimorphism in stature is probably related to sex-biased parental investment influencing nutrition during childhood (Holden and Mace 1999). Female growth spurts occur at a younger age than male growth spurts, and tend to occur before becoming fertile, perhaps because the consequences of pregnancy whilst being underdeveloped would be so serious for girls. In particular, growth in the width of the hips is associated with the onset of fertility (Bogin 1999). Early maturation can also be hazardous for boys; Hill and Hurtado (1996) described how Ache boys are initiated once they start making serious advances towards girls, making them eligible targets in club fights with adult males.

The onset of puberty, which is coincident with the slowing of growth in females, appears to show great plasticity according to environmental circumstances. Stearns and Koella (1986) illustrated how there is neither a fixed height or age at menarche, but a reaction norm exists, where malnourished females will reach menarche at a greater age but a lesser height. A secular trend towards earlier puberty in well-nourished populations has been noted everywhere.

Mating and Marriage

In human societies, mating patterns are frequently legalized in marriage, and marriage patterns are highly diverse. The majority of cultures show patrilocal marital residence (females move from the natal group live with their husbands' family). Seielstad et al. (1998) use genetic evidence – that spatial variability in Y chromosomes appears to be less than in MtDNA or X chromosome – to argue that we are essentially patrilocal; women are more likely to migrate. Our closest primate relatives, chimpanzees and bonobos, show female dispersal, which has been used to argue that patrilocality is ancestral in humans; however, given 5 million years of evolution, and the diversity of marriage patterns within our own species, we should not take this as a certainty. Hunter-gatherers show diverse lineality or no lineality at all, and the origin of defendable and heritable wealth changes everything. A significant minority of human groups show matrilineal descent, where wealth (such as land) is inherited down the female line and mothers live with their daughters, who inherit their fields; marital residence is matrilocal. Men have little in the way of personal possessions, but are meant to pass them on to their sister's children, not their own children (Schneider and Gough 1961). Marriages are typically unstable in matrilineal societies, because a male's investment in his wife's children is low, and therefore the emphasis on marital fidelity is weak. However, the emergence of valuable, heritable wealth, such as livestock, that needs to be defended against theft by men, has been associated with patrilineality (Engels 1884; Aberle 1961; Mace and Holden 1999). Here wealth is passed from father to sons, marital residence is patrilocal and the emphasis on marital fidelity is strong. Wives, frequently purchased with brideprice, become possessions who are not free to leave as they would lose wealth and children if they did.

The extent to which marriage patterns reflect mating patterns is unclear. It is difficult to get direct data on paternity uncertainty in humans for ethical reasons, but several estimates tend to settle at around 10 %. An intriguing method of estimating paternity uncertainty has been used by Gaulin et al. (1997) and Euler and Weitzel (1994), who used kin selection theory (Hamilton 1964) to show that matrilineal relatives invest more in children than patrilineal relatives in western

Europe and the USA in proportions consistent with paternity uncertainty between 9 and 15 %.

Two consistent influences in human mate choice are age and wealth. It is clear from sex differences in fertility through the life course that females should be most in demand as marriage partners when young, but males can achieve high fertility even when quite old (Fig. 1c). The extent to which this is true again depends on the socioeconomic circumstances in which people live. A polygynous marriage system combined with patrilineal ownership of resources (as seen in this Gambian case) means that old men can have young wives if they own the resources to support them and their children. It may be advantageous for young women to marry older, polygynous men if they are wealthier. For example, Josephson (1993) used historical demographic records to show that polygynous Mormon wives in 18th century Utah did have more grandchildren than monogamously married women. Where inherited resources contribute strongly to future reproductive success, marriage can be delayed and competition between siblings can be shown to directly reduce the reproductive success of those inheriting less(Low 1991; Mace 1996a).

The Pace of Childbearing

Reproductive scheduling in human females has characteristics strikingly different from those of other great apes. First, 2.5- to 3-year interbirth intervals appear rather short for our body size (for example, gibbons have 3-year interbirth intervals, chimpanzees 4–5 years, orangutans nearer 8 years). Second, reproduction terminates about halfway through adulthood with menopause, a programmed senescence of the reproductive organs perhaps 20 years before the equivalent senescence is seen in the rest of the body. The biological ability of women to reproduce again after each birth is dictated by a number of energetic influences on ovulation, including breast-feeding patterns and workload (Ellison 1994).

Birth intervals tend to increase with age even before menopause is reached. This may be part of the ageing process, or an evolved response derived from sibling competition. There is evidence from some societies that slowing of reproduction is associated with achieving the desired family size. For example, the absence of a son in the family in a patrilineal society is associated with continued reproduction (e.g., Nath and Land 1994; Mace and Sear 1997).

The relatively rapid pace of childbearing in the first half of adulthood leads to a number of offspring at different stages of dependency, needing to be cared for simultaneously. The ability to achieve such a family has been attributed to mothers being able to co-opt help with childcare and nutrition from other family members. It is possible the male provisioning, which is not seen in other primates, enables high birth rates in human females (Hill 1993), but it has also been argued that post-menopausal females may be the source of that additional, energetic contribution to the family (Hawkes et al. 1997). Whoever was the greatest influence is not agreed upon, but it seems unlikely that raising a human family was a job for mothers alone. Childcare may have been a responsibility for all but the youngest ages, whether as an older sibling, a parent, or a grandparent.

The Evolution of Menopause

Menopause may have evolved precisely so that older women could assist their children reproduce rather than continue to do so themselves, a theory known as the grandmother hypothesis (Williams 1957; Hamilton 1966). If females were dispersing at marriage, then it may be necessary to argue the grandmothers were helping their daughters-in-law rather than their daughters. The genetic relatedness to the child of a daughter-in-law and to the child of a daughter will differ by the extent to which paternity is uncertain. Thus the issue of the evolution of the pace of childbearing and the evolution of menopause are linked with each other, and with the issue of what was our ancestral family structure.

Evidence that women can increase their number of grandchildren by an amount sufficient to outweigh the loss of their own reproductive opportunities is mixed. Simple models have failed to make for-going reproduction in favour of grandmothering appear to be evolutionarily stable (Hill and Hurtado 1991, 1996; Rogers 1993). However, these models are based on the assumption that the risks of reproduction and the benefits of grandmothering have to outweigh the benefits of continued reproduction at the rate of a young woman, which ignores a huge range of costs and benefits that alter with age. Shanley (1999) has developed models of human female life history in which inevitable, generalised biological senescence is included; here the criteria favouring menopause emerge as far less stringent. The risk of maternal mortality is a key parameter in all of these models, because this is what would deprive existing children of maternal care if fertility continued into old age. Maternal mortality risk has generally been assumed to be constant, but in fact it rises *exponentially* with age (Loudon 1992), as does neonatal mortality. Data from maternity hospitals in the USA and the UK in the 1930s show that the causes of maternal death that accelerate with age were not those related to infection but to haemorrhage and placental *praevia,* possibly suggesting a role for reduced muscle strength and tone rather than reduced immunocompetence. In older women, the womb is unable to contract to prevent blood loss as effectively as in younger women, a problem now anticipated with ergometrine injections routinely administered just after delivery. It is possible that the combination of our large babies and the rapid reproductive rate that our social system allows imposes very high risks on continuing reproduction into old age. If these risks were to accelerate further with age, as is not unlikely given the multifactorial nature of ageing, surviving a natural delivery in old age could become highly unlikely and the termination of reproduction by age 50 would need virtually no other explanation.

Hawkes et al. (1997) argued that our reproductive period is not especially short because it fits with a more general primate pattern (Charnov 1993), and that a long post-menopausal life span is the derived character that requires explanation. If true, again, the fitness benefits of grandmothering would not have to be so great for that to evolve (although this argument does not explain why men also have typically similar longevity to women but without male menopause). Hawkes et al. (1997) found that Hadza (forager) children who had a postmenopausal relative in their family group (albeit a very small sample) were fed by them and were better nourished than those that did not. The grandmaternal contribution appeared to be especially important when the child's mother had another baby. They stressed the importance of tubers, which are hard for children to extract and process, and appear to be far more important in the diet than meat. Blurton-Jones et al. (1999) argued that grandmaternal help may be responsible for making early weaning possible in humans.

Quite apart from the risk of maternal mortality discussed above, there are a number of general and specifically human reasons why family sizes should not get too large. Only a small proportion of births are to women over the age of 40 in any society, even though menopause is nearer age 50 (Wood 1994). Both Hill and Hurtado (1996) and Rogers (1993) note that menopause would be much more advantageous if other costs paid by existing children were included. Competition between siblings for parental investment is one such factor. Whilst it is not clear that the effects of sibling competition on mortality are sufficient to curtail reproduction, there may be effects of such competition on future reproductive success that are. Mace (1998) modeled optimal reproductive scheduling when siblings compete for parental wealth, when that wealth influences their future reproductive success. The models showed that it is very rarely optimal for women to have the maximum fertility; thus, over a wide range of realistic cases, the cost of menopause would have been virtually zero. Competition for food, status, territories, breeding opportunities, or kin support could all follow similar dynamics, making large families show diminishing returns. Thus only small biological costs of maintaining female fertility beyond age 50 could favour menopause.

In such circumstances, the benefits of parental and grandparental solicitude would not have to be very great to maintain an extended life span. And the list of possible benefits is long. Figure 2 shows data from the Gambia which suggest just babies born are more likely to survive if their maternal grandmother is alive. This preliminary analysis of the survival of firstborn children suggests that the benefits of a living, maternal grandmother appear after the first 18 months, a pattern that is consistent with the hypothesis that these grandmothers are also contributing to feeding their grandchildren after weaning. Sear et al. (2000) have confirmed that this effect is statistically significant over all birth orders, can be important to the survival of a child in case of the death of its own mother. The long-term benefits of caring for existing daughters could potentially overtake the risk-associated benefits of another late-in-life baby.

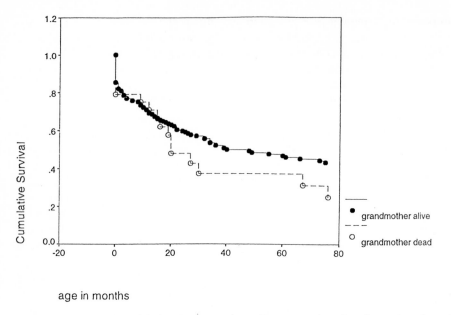

age in months

Fig. 2. Kaplan-Meier plots of the first births to women of known age, from the villages of Keneba and Manduar, between 1968 and 1975. Survival of firstborns, as a function of age in months, according to whether or not their maternal grandmothers were alive at the time of their birth

Conclusion

I have tried to illustrate how approaches from evolutionary ecology contribute to our understanding of our own life history. Whilst it would be tempting to relate all the strange attributes of human life history back to one single effect (such as our big brain, or low adult mortality, or some aspect of our social system or diet), one lesson from studies in life history is that different traits are subject to different selection pressures. It is the combination of selection pressures influencing mortality and fertility that will favour a particular life history strategy, and models reveal that small changes in these selection pressures can have large effects on the optimal life history. Even in closely related species, different trade-offs appear to emerge as important. More studies will reveal the variation across cultures in human life histories, and in the trade-offs that are observed. Over time it will become apparent whether or not any consistent patterns emerge.

Acknowledgements

My research is funded by the Wellcome Trust. Data from The Gambia were collected by Sir Ian McGregor, as part of a long-term collaboration between the MRC and the Gambian government. I thank Rebecca Sear for help preparing the figures, and all those in the Gambia life history research project, Nadine Allal, Tom Kirkwood, Rebecca Sear, Daryl Shanley, Fiona Steele and Andrew Prentice, for helpful discussions, and Richard Sibly for providing helpful comments on the manuscript.

References

Aberle DF (1961) Matrilineal descent in cross-cultural perspective. In: Schneider DM, Gough K (eds) Matrilineal kinshin. Berkely, University of California Press

Alam M (1995) Birth-spacing and infant and early childhood mortality in a high fertility area of Bangladesh – age-dependent and interactive effects. J Biosocial Sci 27:393–404

Barker DJP (1994) Mothers, babies and disease in later life. London, BMJ Publishing Group

Nlurton-Jones N, Hawkes K, O'Connel JF (1999) Some current ideas about evolution of the human life history. In: Lee PC (ed) Comparative primate socioecology. Cambridge, Cambridge University Press

Bogin B (1999) Patterns of human growth. 2nd Edition. Cambridge, Cambridge University Press

Bohler E, Bergstrom S (1995) Subsequent pregnancy effects morbidity of previous child. J Biosocial Sci 27:431–442

Cavalli-Sforza LL, Menozzi P, Piazzo A (1994) The history and geography of human genes. Princeton, Princeton University Press

Charnov EL (1993) Life histroy invariants. Oxford, Oxford University Press

Daly M, Wilson MI (1985) Child abuse and other risks of not living with both parents. Ethol and Sociobiol 6:155–76

Daly M, Wilson MI (1996) Violence against stepchildren. Curr Directions Psychol Sci 5:77–81

DasGupta M (1987) Selective discrimination against female children in rural Punjab. Pop Devel Rev 13:77–100

Ellison PT (1994) Advances in human reproductive ecology. Ann Rev Anthropol 23:255–75

Engels F (1884) The origin of the family, private property and the state. London, Penguin Classics

Euler HA, Weitzel B (1996) Discriminative grandparental solicitude as reproductive strategy. Human Nature 7:39–59

Gaulin SJC, McBurney DH, Brakeman-Wartell SL (1997) Matrilateral biases in the investment of aunts and uncles: a consequence and measure of paternity uncertainty. Human Nature 8:139–151

Graham W (1991) Maternal mortalit levels, trends and data deficiencies. In: Feacham R, Jamison D (eds) Disease and mortality in sub-Saharan Africa. Oxford, Oxford University Press, pp 101–126

Haig D (1999) Genetic conflicts of pregnancy childhood. In: Stearns SC (ed) Evolution in health and disease. Oxford, Oxford University Press, pp 77–89

Hamilton WD (1964) The genetical evolution of social behaviour. J Theoret Biol 7:1–52

Hamilton WD (1966) The moulding of senescence by natural selection.. J Theoret Biol 12:12–45

Harpending HC, Pennington R (1991) Age structure and sex-biased mortality among Herero pastoralists. Human Biol 63:329–353

Hawkes K, O'Connell JF, Blurton-Jones NG (1997) Hadza women's time allocation, offspring provisioning, and the evolution of long post-menopausal lifespans. Curr Anthropol 38:551–578

Hill K (1993) Life history theory and evolutionary anthropology. Evol Anthropol 2:78–88

Hill K, Hurtado AM (1991) The evolution of reproductive senescence and menopause in human females. Human Nature 2:315–350

Hill K, Hurtado AM (1996) Ache life history: the ecology and demography of a foraging people. New York, Aldine de Gruyter

Hobcraft J, McDonald JW, Rutstein S (1983) Child-spacing effects in infant and early child mortality. Pop Index 49:585–618

Holden C, Mace R (1997) A phylogenetic analysis of the evolution of lactose digestion in adults. Human Biol 69:605–628

Holden C, Mace R (1999) Sexual dimorphism in stature and women's work: a cross-cultural analysis. Am J Phys Anthropol 110:27–45

Howell N (1979) Demography of the Dobe area !Kung. New York, Academic Press

Josephson SC (1993) Status, reproductive success and marrying polygynously. Ethol Sociobiol 14:391–396

Kirkwood TBL, Rose MR (1991) Evolution of senescence: late survival sacrificed for reproduction. Phil Trans Roy Soc London B 332;15–24

Lack D (1968) Ecological adaptations for breeding in birds. London, Methuen

LeGrand T, Phillips JF (1996) The effect of fertility reductions on infant and child mortality: evidence from Matlab in rural Bangladesh. Pop Stud 50:51–68

Loudon I (1992) Death in childbirth: an international study of maternal care and maternal mortality 1800–1950. Oxford, Clarendon Press

Low BS (1991) Reproductive life in 19th century Sweden: an evolutionary perspective on demographic phenomena. Ethol Sociobiol 12:411–448

Lund E (1990) Pattern of childbearing and mortality in married women – a national prospective study from Norway. J Epidemiol Commun Health 44:237–240

Mace R (1996a) Biased parental investment and reproductive success in Gabbra pastoralists. Behav Ecol Sociobiol 38:75–81

Mace R (1998) The co-evolution of human fertility and wealth inheritance. Phil Trans Roy Soc London B 353:389–397

Mace R, Sear R (1996) Maternal mortality in a Kenyan, pastoralist population. Intl J Gynecol Obstet 74:137–141

Mace R, Sear R (1997) The birth interval and the sex of children: evidence from a traditional African population. J Biosoc Sci 29:499–507

Mace R, Holden C (1999) Evolutionary ecology and cross-cultural comparison: the case of matrilineality in sub-Saharan Africa. In: Lee PC (ed) Comparative primate socioecology. Cambridge, Cambridge University Press

Moore SE, Coole T, Poski E, Sonko B, Whitehead R, McGregor I, Prentice AM (1997) Season of birth predicts mortality in rural Gambia. Nature 388:434

Nath DC, Land KC (1994) Sex preferences and third birth intervals in a traditional Indian society. J Bioso Sci 26:95–106

Pagel MD, Harvey PH (1989) Taxonomic differences in the scaling of brain weight on body weight among mammals. Science 244:1589–1593

Pennington R (1992) Did food increase fertility? Evaluation of !Kung and Herero history. Human Biol 64:497–521

Perls TT, Alpert L, Fretts RC (1997) Middle-aged mothers live longer. Nature 389:133

Perreira M, Fairbanks LA (1991) Juvenile primates. New York & Oxford, Oxford University Press

Roff DA (1992) The evolution of life histories: theory and analysis. London, Chapman & Hall

Rogers AR (1993) Why menopause? Evol Ecol 7:406–420

Scheper-Hughes N (1992) Death without weeping: the violence of everyday life in Brazil. Berkely, University of California Press

Schneider DM, Gough K (1961) Matrilineal kinship. Berkeley, University of California Press

Sear R, Mace R, McGregor IA (2000) Maternal grandmothers improve nutritional status and survival of children in rural Gambia. Proc Roy Soc Lond B 267:1–7

Seielstad MT, Minch E, Cavalli-Sforza LL (1998) Genetic evidence for higher female migration rate in humans. Nature Genet 20:278–288

Shanley D (1999) Resources, reproduction and senescence: evolutionary optimality models. Unpublished Ph.D. thesis. University of Manchester

Simoons FJ (1978) The geographic hypothesis and lactose malabsorption: a weighing of the evidence. Am J Digest Diseases 23:963–980

Stearns SC (1992) The evolution of life histories. Oxford, Oxford University Press

Stearns SC, Koella J (1986) The evolution of phenotypic plasticity in life history traits: predictions for norms of reaction for age- and size-at-maturity. Evolution 40:893–913

Strassman B, Dunbar RLM (1999) Human evolution and disease: putting the Stone Age in perspective. In: Stearns SC (ed) Evolution in health and disease. Oxford, Oxford University Press, pp 91–101

Symons D (1979) The evolution of human sexuality. Oxford, Oxford University Press

Tracer D (1991) Fertility related changes in maternal body composition among the Au of Papua New Guinea. Am J Phys Anthropol 85:393–406

Voland E (1988) Differential infant and child mortality in evolutionary perspective: data from late 17th to 19th century Ostfriesland (Germany). In: Betzig L et al. (eds) Human reproductive behaviour – a Darwinian perspective. Cambridge, Cambridge University Press

Williams GC (1957) Pleiostropy, natural selection and the evolution of senescence. Evolutions 11:398–411

Westendorp R, Kirkwood TBL (1998) Human longevity at the cost of reproductive success. Nature 396:743–746

Wood JW (1994) Dynamics of human reproduction: biology, demography. New York, Aldine de Gruyter

Caretaking, Risk-seeking, and Survival in Anthropoid Primates

J. Allman and A. Hasenstaub

Animals with big brains are rare. If brains enable animals to adapt to changing environments, why is it that so few animals have large brains? The answer is that large brains are very expensive, both in terms of the energy needed to support them and the long time needed for them to mature (Allman 1998; Allman and Hasenstaub 1999). Thus the rearing of large-brained offspring requires parental support for commensurately long periods. Moreover, large-brained offspring are mostly single births and the interbirth intervals are long, which also reflect the large costs of rearing these offspring. The parents must live long enough past their sexual maturity to sustain the serial production and maintenance of a sufficient number of offspring to replace themselves while allowing for the early death or infertility of their offspring. If the caretaking parent dies, the orphan will have a high probability of dying as well, but if the non-caretaking parent dies, this event will have little impact on the offspring's chances of survival. Therefore, we hypothesized that, in large-brained species that have single births, the sex that bears the greater burden in providing care for offspring will tend to survive longer. Genes enhancing the survival of the caretaking parent will be favored by natural selection since they will be more likely to be transmitted to the next generation than genes enhancing the survival of the noncaretaking parent. Male primates are incapable of gestating infants and lactating; but in several species, fathers carry and feed their offspring for long periods, and the young may stay close to the father even after they move independently. According to the caretaking theory, females should live longer than males in the species where the mother does most or all of the care of offspring, there should be no difference in survival between the sexes in species in which both parents participate about equally in infant care, and in those few species where the father does a greater amount of care than the mother, males should live longer. We tested this hypothesis by constructing mortality tables for male and female anthropoids (monkeys, apes and humans) based on studbook records from captive populations and comparing these data with the sexual division of care for offspring (Allman et al. 1998).

The great apes are our closest relatives. Chimpanzees, orangutans and gorillas nearly always give birth to a single offspring and the interval between births ranges from 4 to 8 years. Female chimpanzees, orangutans, and gorillas have a large survival advantage in data obtained from captive populations. For example, in captivity the average male chimpanzee lives about 67 % as long as the average female (see Table 1; Dyke et al. 1995). In the case of chimpanzees there also are

Robine et al. (Eds.)
Sex and Longevity: Sexuality, Gender,
Reproduction, Parenthood
© Springer-Verlag Berlin Heidelberg 2000

Table 1. The ratio of average male to female life span and patterns of parental care for anthropoid primates (Allman et al. 1998). The right column is the index of sexual dimorphism: the ratio of average male to female body weight. The body weight data were kindly provided by Professor Bob Martin

Primate	Male/female survival ratio	Male care			Male/Female weight ratio
Titi monkey	1.208	Carries infant from birth	↑		1.139
Owl monkey	1.151	Carries infant from birth			1.026
Siamang	1.093	Carries infant in second year	Increasing Male Survival		1.279
Goeldi's monkey	1.027	Both parents carry infant		Increasing Male Care	1.000
Human (Sweden 1780–1991)	0.924–0.951	Supports economically, some care			1.182
Gorilla	0.889	Protects, plays with offspring			1.851
Gibbon	0.834	Pair-living, but little direct role			1.044
Orangutan	0.831	None			2.095
Spider monkey	0.786	Rare or negligible			1.001
Chimpanzee	0.667	Rare or negligible			1.355

data available from natural populations. In her longterm study of the chimpanzees of Gombe in Tanzania, Goodall found that adult males died at a higher rate than females (Goodall 1986). In a 22-year study of a population of 228 chimpanzees living in the Mahale Mountains near the shores of Lake Tanganyika, Nishida (1990) found an equivalent number of male and female births but three times as many females as males in the adult population. This difference was not due to differential patterns of migration, and thus these observations indicate a strong female survival advantage for chimpanzees living in the wild. Chimpanzee mothers generally provide nearly all the care for their offspring, and females possess a very strong survival advantage. Although male care of infants is rare in chimpanzees, Goodall (1986) and Pascal Gagneux and colleagues (1999) have observed instances in which males have adopted orphaned infants and cared for them. Their observations indicate that the potential for male care is present in chimpanzees, though rarely expressed. The maternal dependency is indicated by Nishida's (1990) observation that the death of the mother is a leading cause of death in young chimpanzees. Goodall (1986) found that about half of orphaned chimpanzees died and that the surviving orphans often exhibited retarded sexual maturation. Maternal support is also linked to the success of adult offspring in chimpanzees (Goodall 1986; Nishida 1990), and this is probably another factor favoring the evolution of survival-enhancing genes in chimpanzees.

Orangutan mothers provide all the care for their offspring, which have very little contact with the solitary adult males (Rodman and Mitani 1987). We found that male orangutans live about 83 % as long as females (see Fig. 1 and Table 1). Gorilla mothers provide most of the care for their offspring, but the fathers protect and play with them. The female survival advantage in gorillas, while significant, is not so large as in chimpanzees or orangutans.

The lesser apes are our next closest relatives. Gibbons and siamangs live in pairs and have a single baby about once every three years. They maintain their

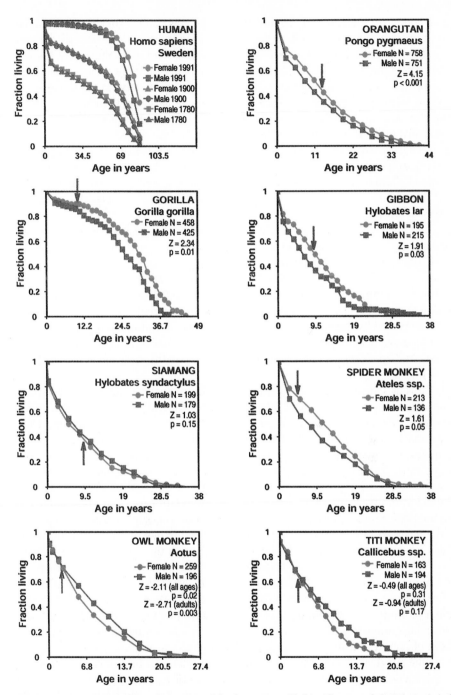

Fig. 1. Primate survival tables. The sources of the data are provided in Allman et al. (1998). Statistical significance was measured using Gehan's generalized Wilcoxon test (Lee 1992). The arrows indicate the average age at which females have their first offspring

pair bonds and defend their territories through spectacular vocalizations similar to the pair-bonding songs of birds. Gibbon mothers provide nearly all the care for their offspring, but Chivers (1974) found that siamang fathers play a much larger parental role than do gibbon fathers. Siamang mothers carry their infants for the first year, but during the second year the father mostly carries the growing infant. Siamang fathers are unique among apes in carrying their infants and in the closeness of their bonding with their offsprings. Gibbon females have a survival advantage over males, but the situation is reversed in siamangs, where the males have a small advantage. Gibbons males on average live about 83 % percent as long as females, but siamang males live 9 % longer than females (see Fig. 1 and Table 1). Siamangs are the only apes in which fathers regularly carry their infants for substantial periods of time and the only apes in which females do not have a survival advantage.

In Old World monkeys, females do most of the infant care. Female survival advantages have been reported in studies of mortality in natural populations of two species. In Toque macaques (*Macaca sinica*), females older than four years have a lower risk of dying than males of comparable age (Dittus 1977). In gelada baboons (*Theropithecus gelada*), females older than 8.5 years have a lower risk of dying than males of the same age (Dunbar 1980). A female survival advantage is also suggested by the substantial female majorities found in adult populations of all 12 species of cercopithecine monkeys (baboons, macaques, verveta), that have been studied demographically under natural conditions (Melnick and Pearl 1987).

In New World monkeys, we found a significant survival advantage in captive spider monkeys (see Fig. 1 and Table 1). Females constitute the majority of adults in all of natural populations of spider monkeys that have been studied (Van Roosmalen and Klein 1988). There are typically about 30 percent more adult females than males in spider monkey groups. In his demographic study of mortality rates, Robinson (1988) found a female survival advantage in a large natural population of capuchin monkeys that he studied in Venezuela. In both spider and capuchin monkeys, mothers do virtually all the infant care (Van Roosmalen and Klein 1988; Freese and Oppenheimer 1981). However, the situation is dramatically reversed in two other New World primates, the owl monkeys and titi monkeys. These monkeys live in monogamous pairs with their young. In her study of owl monkey and titi monkey families living under natural conditions in Peru, Wright (1984) found that the fathers carry their infants from almost immediately after birth except for brief nursing periods on the mother and occasional rides on older siblings. She also found that the fathers frequently shared food with their offspring, something the mothers rarely did. In our colony of owl monkeys, we have observed that, if the father dies, the mother will not carry the infant, and thus the survival of the infant depends on the father. In both owl and titi monkeys, males and females die at the same rate until maturity, but after maturity the males have a survival advantage over females. Thus the timing of the male survival advantage corresponds to the period in their lives when they carry their offspring. Although owl monkeys and titi monkeys are similar in size, monogamy, and parenting behavior, DNA sequence data indicate that they are not closely related genetically (Schneider and Rosenberger 1996; Porter et al. 1999). Thus extensive paternal care with enhanced male survival is a specialization that probably evolved independently in lines leading to modern owl monkeys and titi monkeys.

Another New World monkey, *Callimico goeldi*, lives in small groups with more than one adult male and female in each group. In Goeldi's monkeys, births are single. The mother carries the infant for the first three weeks, but subsequently adult males carry it in cooperation with other family members (Kinzey 1997). The postnatal care provided by each sex is roughly equivalent and is distributed throughout the group. We found nearly identical survival curves for males and females (see Table 1 and Allman et al. 1998). Goeldi's monkeys also have accelerated maturation, with first reproduction occurring at about 1.3 years, far earlier than any other monkey, and females have two birth seasons per year (Kinzey 1997). However, Goeldi's monkeys are not shorter lived than other primates of their body weight (Hakeem et al. 1996). Goeldi's monkeys were formerly classified within their own family of New World monkeys, but more recent studies have placed them within the callithricids with the marmosets and tamarins (Schneider and Rosenberger 1996). Unlike other monkeys, marmosets and tamarins usually give birth to twins or sometimes triplets. Shortly after birth, females become sexually receptive and can conceive again. Thus marmosets and tamarin females can produce up to six infants per year. These primates have developed a different way to care for their multiple, slowly developing, large-brained infants. Marmosets and tamarins live in extended families in which everyone, and especially the adult males, participate in infant care. There is typically more than one adult male per family, and they cooperate in infant care (Garber 1997). Because of the cooperative care, offspring are not dependent on the survival of a particular caretaker. In our preliminary studies in marmosets and tamarins, we have found little difference in the survival of males and females. Through intensely cooperative care of infants, callithricids have overcome the evolutionary constraints imposed by large brain size and slow development (Allman 1998).

It is well known that women tend to live longer than men. It is often assumed that this is a modern phenomenon resulting from the greatly reduced risk of death in childbirth. However, the female survival advantage is present in the oldest systematic records from a human population, which were collected in Sweden beginning in 1780, long before modern health practices were instituted. The female advantage is present at every age and for every Swedish census since 1780 (Keyfitz and Flieger 1968–1990). In the Swedish population women live 5 to 8 % longer than men. Similar female advantages were recorded in the earliest data from England and France in the 19th century and a female advantage has been present in most nations throughout the world in the 20th century (Keyfitz and Flieger 1968–1990). According to current World Health Organization (1998) data, females live longer than males in all but two of 171 reporting countries (see Fig. 2). A female survival advantage has also been found for adults in the Ache, a well-studied hunter-gatherer population living in the forests of eastern Paraguay

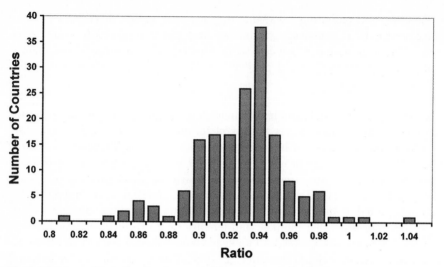

Fig. 2. Histogram of the ratios of average male life expectancy to female life expectancy for 171 countries. The graph was constructed from data from the World Health Organization (1998)

(Hill and Hurtado 1996). These data indicate that the survival advantage in human females has deep biological roots. However, it is smaller relative to life span than in chimpanzees, spider monkeys, orangutans, gibbons, arid gorillas (see Table 1).

In most species there is a female advantage throughout life, but in all the anthropoid primates in which there are single births and the males carry their offspring, there is either no difference in survival between the sexes or there is a definite male survival advantage (see Table 1). These results run counter to the expectation that lugging a heavy squirming infant through the trees would increase the risk of disease or injury to the caretaker. The magnitude of the difference in survival corresponds to the difference in the amount of care given to the offspring by each sex. Thus in the great apes, where the mothers do most of the care, there is a large female advantage. Human males contribute significantly, but human females are the primary caregivers, and in humans there is a proportionally smaller, but still sizable female advantage. In Goeldi's monkeys both sexes provide about the same amount of care and there is no difference in survival. In callithricids, there is a large amount of cooperation within the extended family in carrying and sharing food with the offspring, which reduces the dependency on any particular caretaker. In siamangs, both parents participate with the father taking over in the later stages of infant development, and siamang males have a small advantage. In owl monkeys and titi monkeys, males carry the infants from almost immediately from birth, and thus infant survival depends substantially on the male; in these monkeys there is a large male survival advantage.

Darwin (1874) proposed that large male body size was related to male competition, and therefore the ratio of male to female body weight has been seen as an indicator of the intensity of male competition (Dixson 1999). We examined the relationship between the male/female body weight ratio with the male/female survival ratio under the premise that male fighting might account for some of the differences in male mortality among primates. In Table 1, there is a slight tendency for the male/female survival ratio to be negatively related to the male/female body weight ratio but the effect is not significant ($R^2 = 0.12$; $p = 0.37$). This tendency is not seen in the two most closely related primates in the table, gibbons and siamangs, where it is the more sexually dimorphic siamangs that exhibit male care and a higher male/female survival ratio. In addition, spider monkey males and females are the same size, but males live only about 79 % as long as females. Thus the pattern of sex differences in survival cannot be accounted for by sexual dimorphism as a measure of male competition.

In the contemporary United States population, females have lower mortality rates than males for the 13 most prevalent causes of death, which indicates that the female survival advantage has an extremely broad base (Anderson et al. 1997). A higher incidence of smoking in men may contribute to this effect, but among non-smokers aged 35 to 69, men have a 41 % higher mortality rate than women (Peto et al. 1994). A probable hormonal basis for the lower female mortality rate is evidenced by the finding by Grodstein and her collaborators (1997) that post-menopausal women who currently receive estrogen replacement have a lower risk of death as compared to post-menopausal women who have never received supplemental estrogen.

Another possible basis for differential survival may be related to the stress hormones, the corticosteroids. The clearest evidence for this comes from a study by Sapolsky (1992) done in vervets, Old World monkeys in which females provide most of the care for offspring. In a group of vervets that had been subjected to chronic stress due to living in crowded conditions, Sapolsky (1992) found a substantial loss of neurons in part of the hippocampus, in males but not in females. The hippocampal neurons are richly supplied with receptors for the corticosteroid hormones, which are produced by the adrenal cortex to mobilize the body's defenses when subjected to stress. One role of the hippocampus is to regulate the pituitary's secretion of adrenocorticotropic hormone, which in turns signals the adrenal cortex to secrete the corticosteriod hormones into the blood stream. Secretion of the corticosteroid hormones is the body's way of responding to severe, life-threatening situations, but chronic secretion of these hormones can be very damaging. The hippocampal neurons are particularly vulnerable because they have many receptors for these hormones. The loss of the hippocampal neurons eliminates the negative feedback on the secretion of the stress hormones thus leading to escalating levels of damage and ultimately to death. Sapolsky's (1992) results indicate that male vervets are much more vulnerable to the destruction of the brain's system for regulating the stress response than are females. This may be the mechanism for male vulnerability in other species where females are the primary caregivers, and the opposite may be true for those species where males are the primary caregivers.

The differential mortality between caretakers and noncaretakers may be in part because the former are risk-averse and the latter tend to be risk-seeking

(Allman 1998). Risk-seekers constantly probe their world, seeking out new opportunities and detecting hazards in the constantly changing environment. Through their probing they generate new information that they communicate to close kin, thus enhancing their kin's survival and the propagation of their shared genes. Caretakers tend to avoid risk because they risk not only themselves but also their offspring. This may be a conscious decision or may be the result of genetically determined instincts that would be favored by natural selection because they would lead to more surviving offspring. A second major factor may be a differential vulnerability to the damaging effects of stress. Natural selection would also favor the evolution of genes in caretakers that protect them against the damage induced by stress. The ratio between the rates at which males and female die varies during the course of life. In humans, the female survival advantage begins shortly after conception and continues throughout life, with the largest advantage, in terms of the size of the ratio between male and female age-specific death rates, occurring at around age 25 (see Fig. 3). In many countries there is evidence for a second, smaller peak or shoulder in the male to female death ratios later in life. Although smaller, these two peaks have been present in the Swedish population since 1780 (Keyfitz and Flieger 1968). They also are present in young and late adulthood in some nonhuman primates such as chimpanzees and gorillas (Herndon et al. 1999; Allman et al. 1998). The increase in amplitude of these peaks in human populations since about 1950 is probably due to decreased mortality from infectious diseases in which the female survival advantage is typically smaller than for other causes of death. For example, for septicemia the ratio of the male mortality rate to the female rate is only 1.2 to 1, which is nearer to parity than for most of the other major causes of death in the United States (Anderson et al. 1997).

The peak in early adulthood corresponds approximately to the period of greatest responsibility for childcare in women. The second peak appears to be related to a higher risk of death from various chronic diseases in men. We believe that these two peaks represent two underlying classes of mechanisms, one of which is mainly acting on the young and the other on the old. The first peak is largely due to differences between males and females in risk-taking behavior, which results in higher death rates due to accidents and violence in younger males (see Fig. 4). The second peak may result from increased male vulnerability to pathological conditions that develop without overt symptoms over a long period of time, such as genetic damage ultimately leading to cancer, as well as high blood pressure and arterial plaque build up, all of which may be related to the cumulative effects of stress. Note in Figures 5, 6 and 7 how excess male deaths from heart disease, stroke and cancer pass like waves through age cohorts with similar patterns in different countries. The ratio of male to female death rates from ischemic heart disease peaks at about age 50, for stroke at about age 60, and for cancer at about age 70. Even in a population of hunter-gatherers, Ache women in their 50s and 60s have a lower mortality rate than men, indicating that the female advantage is not solely due to modern health practices (Hill and Hurtado 1996). These deaths from heart disease, stroke, and cancer are mostly occurring

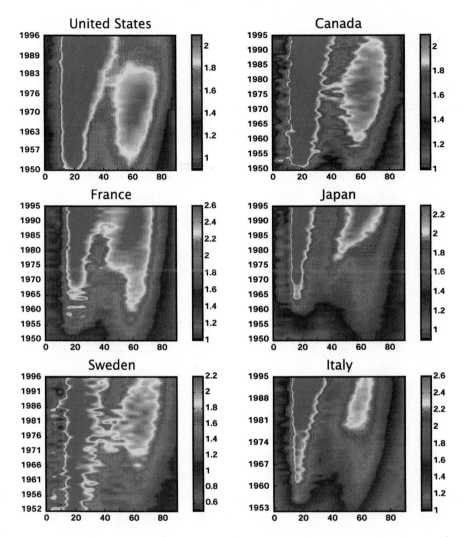

Fig. 3. Male-to-female age-specific mortality ratios. The horizontal axis represents age in years, the vertical axis represents calendar year, and the color plotted is the ratio of the male age-specific mortality rate to the female age-specific mortality rate for the same age and year. Higher age-specific mortality ratios, represented by colors closer to red, indicate ages and years for which the male risk of death exceeds the female risk of death. Raw data were provided by the World Health Organization (http://www.who.int/whosis/mort/download.htm); data analysis was conducted by the authors using Matlab and Perl

past the age of parental care, but reflect sex differences in cumulative damage during that phase of life. The female mortality advantage in late adulthood may also be related to the female role in caring for grandchildren, which would enhance their survival and ultimately the propagation of their grandmother's genes (Hawkes et al. 1998).

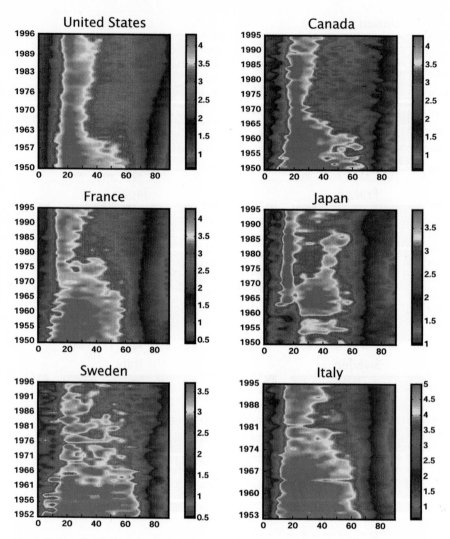

Fig. 4. Male-to-female age-specific mortality ratios for deaths due to murder, suicide, and accidents (ICD 7 categories A138–A150, ICD 8 Categories A138–A150, ICD 9 categories B47–B56). A curious exception to the pattern is the depressed rate of violent deaths in the young adult Japanese males from 1950 to 1960. We speculate that this anomaly may be due to historical reasons associated with the aftermath of the second world war

An examination of the web of relationships between the evolution of large brain size, the long period of postnatal maturation, and the differential roles of caretakers and risk-seekers contributes a new perspective regarding sex- and age-specific patterns of vulnerability to many human afflictions. Large-brained, slow-developing, long-dependent offspring require long-surviving parents to reach maturity. A measure of this parental dependency effect is the differential survival of caretakers versus noncaretakers. In anthropoid primates, the caretaker effect

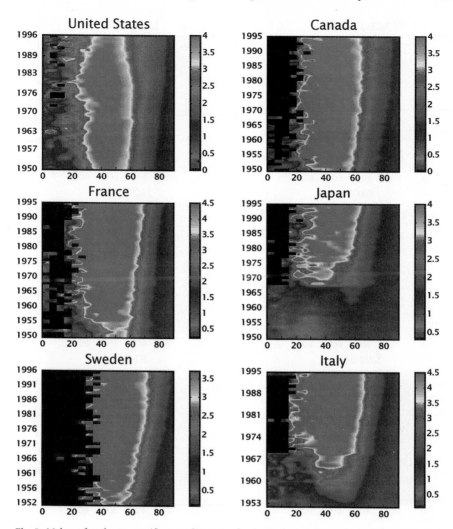

Fig. 5. Male-to-female age-specific mortality ratios for deaths from ischemic heart disease (ICD 7 Category A081, ICD 8 Category A083, ICD 9 Category B27). The anomalous patterns in the Japanese and Italian data prior to 1969 appear to be caused by inconsistent categorization of some heart disease deaths under ICD 7. The irregular pattern in early ages is due to the low incidence of heart disease in young people. Note that although the death rate from ischemic heart disease in the United States dropped 60 % between 1950 and 1996 (Cardiovascular Health Bureau 1999), the male-female mortality differential remained remarkably constant over the same time period

appears to have a large influence on the patterns of survival. Average male life span can be as short as 67 % of female life span in primates where males have negligible roles in caring for offspring versus as much as a 20 % male survival advantage when males carry offspring from soon after birth and share food with them. The male caretaking effect is not as large as for females because only females provide nutrition for their slowly developing offspring through lactation.

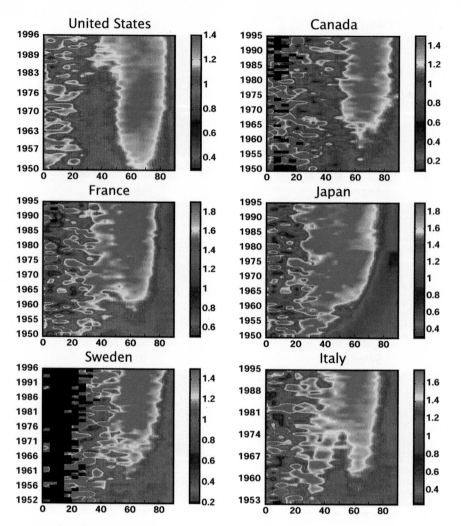

Fig. 6. Male-to-female age-specific mortality ratios for deaths due to stroke (ICD 7 category A070, ICD 8 Category A085, ICD 9 Category B29). The irregular pattern in early ages is due to the low incidence of stroke in young people

We believe that these effects came about mainly through the enhancement of genes favoring caretaker survival through natural selection. The mechanisms responsible for the survival differences between caretakers and noncaretakers may ultimately be related to neurochemical differences that favor risk-averse behavior in caretakers and risk-seeking behavior in noncaretakers, as well as greater vulnerability to chronic diseases resulting from the more damaging effects of stress on noncaretakers.

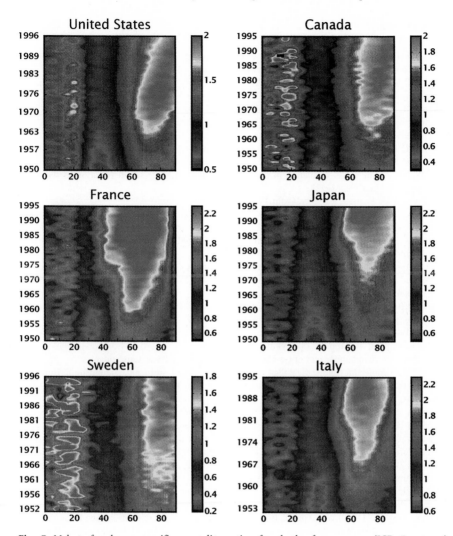

Fig. 7. Male-to-female age-specific mortality ratios for deaths from cancer (ICD 7 categories A044–A060, ICD 8 categories A045–A061, ICD 9 categories B08–B17

Acknowledgements

This research was supported by the Hixon Fund and by the Howard Hughes Medical Institute.

References

Allman JM (1998) Evolving brains. Scientific American Library, New York

Allman J, Hasenstaub A (1999) Brains, maturation times, and parenting. Neurobiol Aging 20:447–454

Allman JM, Rosin A, Kumar R, Hasenstaub A (1998) Parenting and survival in anthropoid primates: caretakers live longer. Proc Natl Acad Sci 95:6866–6869

Anderson R, Kochanek K, Murphy S (1997) Monthly vital statistics report 45:1–80

Cardiovascular Health Bureau (1999) Decline in deaths from heart disease and stroke – United States, 1900–1999. Morbid Mortal Weekly Rep 48:649–656

Chivers D (1974) The siamang in Malaysia. Contrib Primatol 4:1–335

Darwin C (1874) The descent of man. Second edition, Merrill and Baker, New York

Dittus W (1977) The social regulation of population density and age-sex distribution in the toque monkey. Behaviour 63:281–322

Dixson AF (1999) Primate sexuality, Oxford University Press, Oxford

Dunbar R (1980) Demographic and life history variables of a population of gelada baboons (Theropithecus gelada) J Anim Ecol 49:485–506

Dyke B, Gage T, Alford P, Swenson B, Williams-Bangero S (1995) A model lifetable for chimpanzees. Am J Primatol 37:25–37

Freese C, Oppenheimer J (1981) The capuchin monkeys, genus Cebus. In: Coimbra-Filho A, Mittermeier R (eds.) Ecology and behavior of neotropical primates. Vol. 1. Academia Brasileira de Ciencias, Rio de Janeiro, pp 331–390

Gagneux P, Boesch C, Woodruff D (1999) Female reproductive strategies, paternality, and community structure in wild West African chimpanzees. Anim Behav 57:19–32

Garber P (1997) One for all and breeding for one: cooperation and competition as a tamarin reproductive strategy. Evol Anthropol 5:187–199

Goodall J (1986) The chimpanzees of Gombe. Harvard University Press, Cambridge

Grodstein F, Stampfer M, Colditz G, Willett W, Manson J, Joffe M, Rosner B, Hankinson S, Hunter D, Hennekens CH, Speizer FE (1997) Postmenopausal hormone therapy and mortality. New Engl Med 336:1769–1775

Hakeem A, Sandoval G, Jones M, Allman J (1996) Brain and life span in primates. In: Birren J, Schaie W (eds.) Handbook of the psychology of aging. Academic Press, San Diego, pp 78–104

Hawkes K, O'Connell N, Blurton-Jones H, Alvarez H, Charnov E (1998) Grandmothering, menopause, and the evolution of humans life histories. Proc Natl Acad Sci 95:1336–1339

Herndon J, Tigges J, Anderson D, Klumpp S, McClure H (1999) Brain weight throughout the life span of the chimpanzee. J Comp Neurol 409:567–572

Hill K, Hurtado AM (1996) Ache life history. Aldine de Gruyter, New York

Keyfitz N, Flieger W (1968) World population. University of Chicago Press, Chicago

Keyfitz N, Flieger W (1990) World population growth and aging. University of Chicago Press, Chicago

Kinzey WG (1997) New World primates: ecology, evolution, and behavior. Aldine de Gruyter, New York

Lee ET (1992) Statistical methods for survival data analysis. Wiley, New York

Melnick D, Pearl M (1986) Cercopithecines in multimale groups: genetic diversity and population structure. In: Smuts BB, Cheney DL, Seyfarth RM, Wrangham RW, Struhsaker TT (eds) Primate societies. University of Chicago Press, Chicago, pp 121–134

Nishida T (1990) The chimpanzees of the Mahale Mountains. University of Tokyo Press, Tokyo

Peto R, Lopez A, Boreham J, Thun M, Heath C (1994) Mortality for smoking in developed countries 1950–2000. Oxford University Press, Oxford

Porter CA, Czelusniak J, Scheinder H, Schneider MPC, Sampaio I, Goodman M (1999) Sequences from the 5' flanking region of the episilon-globin gene support the relationship of Callicebus with the pithecines. Am J Primatol 48:69–75

Robinson J, Wright P, Kinzey W (1986) Monagamous cebids and their relatives. In: Smuts B, Cheney D, Seyfarth R, Wrangham R, Struhsaker T (eds) Primate Societies. Chicago, University of Chicago Press, pp 69–82

Rodman PS, Mitani JC (1987) Orangutans: sexual dimorphism in a solitary species. In: Smuts BB, Cheney DL, Seyfarth RM, Wrangham RW, Struhsaker TT (eds) Primate societies. University of Chicago Press, Chicago, pp 146154

Sapolsky R (1992) Stress, the aging brain, and the mechanisms of neuron death. MIT Press, Cambridge

Schneider H, Rosenberger AL (1996) Molecules, morphology, and platyrrhine systematics. In: Norconk MA, Rosenberger AL, Garber, PA (eds) Adaptive radiations of neotropical/primates. Plenum, New York, pp 3–19

Van Roosmalen M, Klein, L (1988) The spider monkey, genus Ateles. In: Mittermeier R, Coimbra-Filho A, Fonseca G (eds) Ecology and behavior of neotropical primates. Vol. 2. World Wildlife Fund, Washington, pp 455–537

World Health Organization (1998) The world health report, 1998. World Health Organization, Geneva

Wright, PC (1984) Biparental care in *Aotus trivirgatus* and Callicebus moloch. In: Small M (ed) Female primates. Liss, New York, pp 59–75

The Ecology of Menopause

C. Packer

Abstract

Reproductive senescence is a universal characteristic of mammalian females. In some species, however, reproductive senescence occurs close to midlife, and several theories have been proposed to explain how menopause might be adaptive, especially through fitness benefits to a female's grandchildren. Recent research has clarified how menopause can evolve in the absence of such indirect benefits and instead focuses attention on an aging female's abilities as a mother rather than as a grandmother.

Two alternative paradigms have been developed to explain the evolution of menopause. First, menopause occurs at an age where most females have already died due to disease or predation, and thus selection has become too weak to prevent the expression of deleterious genetic traits that were either neutral or beneficial at younger ages (Williams 1957; Hamilton 1966; Charlesworth 1980). Second, menopause is an adaptation that releases elderly females from the costs of further childbirth (Williams 1957; Rogers 1993) or otherwise enables them to redirect their nurturance to grandchildren (Hawkes et al. 1997).

Menopause is often considered unique to humans, but reproductive cessation is virtually ubiquitous in female mammals (Finch 1990; vom Saal et al. 1994). But even though senescence is inevitable (and therefore provides a reasonable explanation for the origins of menopause), it has been difficult to explain why women's reproduction deteriorates so much earlier than somatic function (Hill and Hurtado 1991). However, any analysis of the human menopause is hampered by the difficulties in establishing relevant life tables in the face of modern agriculture, medicine and sanitation. Madame Calment lived 70–80 years beyond menopause, but would she even have reached the age of 50 in a pre-technological society? Nevertheless, many researchers remain impressed by the apparently young age of the human menopause, and thus the grandmother hypothesis retains considerable popular appeal (e.g., Sherman 1998; Angier 1999; Sapolsky and Finch 1999) despite serious theoretical difficulties (Rogers 1993) and little empirical support (e.g., Hill and Hurtado 1991).

Our recent research on wild populations of African lions and olive baboons (Packer et al. 1998) reinforces the suggestion that reproductive senescence can evolve purely from the force of extrinsic mortality: female lions start breeding by

Robine et al. (Eds.)
Sex and Longevity: Sexuality, Gender, Reproduction, Parenthood
© Springer-Verlag Berlin Heidelberg 2000

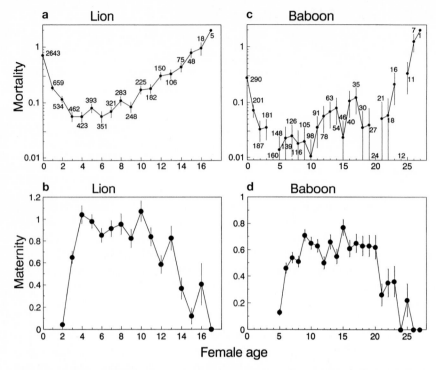

Fig. 1. Age-specific mortality and maternity in female lions and baboons. Bars represent standard errors; numbers are sample size. Annual mortality is estimated from monthly intervals for a, lions (652 yearlings, 18.4 % censored) and from weekly intervals for c, baboons (201 yearlings, 60.7 % censored). Gross maternity for b, lions and d, baboons is the number of live offspring produced at each age

the age of three to four years, suffer an annual mortality of at least 8 %, and undergo an abrupt decline in reproductive rate at the age of 14 (Fig. 1 a,b). Female baboons start breeding by the age of seven to eight years, when annual mortality is only about 2 %, and they show an abrupt drop in reproduction at the age of 21 (Fig. 1 c,d).

Although it is difficult to specify the factors that contribute to declining reproduction in female lions, cycling and fertility are easily measured in baboons. During the menstrual cycle, the perineal sex skin undergoes a distinct tumescence during the follicular phase and a sudden detumescence at the onset of the luteal phase, and the perineum turns scarlet shortly after conception (Altmann 1970). In the Gombe baboons, pregnancies were more likely to end in miscarriage at the age of 21, cycles became more irregular at the age of 23, and fertility essentially stopped by the age of 24 (Fig. 2).

Captive baboons at the Southwest Foundation for Biomedical Research (SFBR) experience a slightly earlier onset of reproductive decline than the Gombe baboons. AT SFBR, females show a striking decrease in cycling regularity by the age of 20–23 and a drop in fertility by the age of 20 (with a complete cessa-

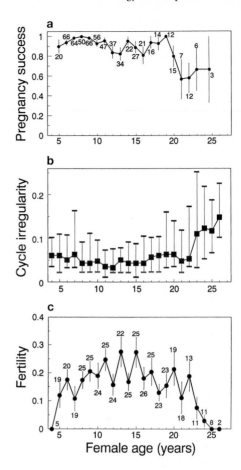

Fig. 2. Age-specific aspects of female reproduction. a, Proportion of baboon pregnancies that ended in live birth. b, Median (■) and quartile (–) "irregularity" of menstrual cycles (irregularity = standardized deviation from the average cycle length, see Packer et al. 1998 for details). c, Mean proportion of cycles resulting in pregnancy (plotted with standard errors and the number of cycling females at each age). Cycles become significantly more irregular while pregnancy success and fertility decline at advanced ages

tion in fertility by the age of 24), and 23 to 29-year-old females secrete far higher levels of follicular stimulating hormone (FSH; Ledford 1998). Such high levels of FSH provide a clear indication of deteriorating ovarian function and eventual menopause, and these same animals also show signs of osteoporosis once they reach their twenties (Lauerman et al. 1992).

Do these patterns reflect age-specific selection pressures in nature? Because of high mortality patterns in both lions and baboons, relatively few females survive long enough to suffer from declining reproductive performance. We estimated the strength of selection for lions to be only 0.0026 at the age of 14 years and 0.0015 for 21-year-old baboons, values which might indeed be too weak to eliminate traits that only harm such elderly individuals.

While this interpretation is reasonably consistent with the traditional view of reproductive senescence, female lions live to a maximum age of 18 in the wild and female baboons live to 27+. Thus reproduction starts to deteriorate well before the end of life. Can this "early" onset of reproductive senescence be due to the value of grandmaternal care in these species?

Lions and baboons would seem like ideal candidates for a "grannie effect" since they both live in complex matrilineal societies. Lions are communal breeders that will even nurse each others' offspring (Packer and Pusey 1997); baboons form kin-based alliances that determine their descendants' dominance ranks (Gouzoules and Gouzoules 1987). However, we found no evidence that grandmother lions or baboons actually enhanced the survival of their grandchildren, except when lion grandmothers were reproductively active (Fig. 3). Lion mothers rear their cubs in communal crèches, whereas non-mothers are relatively asocial (Pusey and Packer 1994). Thus grandmothers only help their grandchildren when they are reproductively active, and menopause not only costs further direct reproduction but also eliminates the opportunity to nurture their grandchildren.

Alternatively, if the mortality risks of parturition increased sufficiently with advancing age, menopause would extend a female's life expectancy long enough to "fledge" her older dependent offspring (Nesse and Williams 1994). However, this suggestion does not apply to lions or baboons since they do not resume breeding until their prior offspring have reached independence (see below). Furthermore, parturition is not a significant source of mortality in either species even at advanced ages (Packer et al. 1998).

Although maternal survival may not enhance the fitness of their early-born offspring, females will receive no genetic return from their final infant if they die before it is fledged. The interbirth interval is about two years in both species, and lions and baboons suffer high mortality if they are orphaned before the age of two years (Fig. 4). Even if the only individual that suffers from the demise of its mother is the last-born offspring, a long period of infant dependency will nevertheless be expected to influence the timing of reproductive senescence.

Figure 5 shows a hypothetical survival curve with constant mortality. Assume that selection is too weak to prevent the fixation of harmful alleles beyond the age where only 1 % of females are still alive (at the age of 10 years). Assume, too, that a mother rears each brood sequentially, waiting until her prior brood has reached two years of age (and can therefore survive on its own) before giving birth to her next brood. When infant survival depends entirely on maternal care, females will gain no further fitness from any reproduction after the age of eight years.

Thus reproductive senescence will inevitably precede somatic senescence, and the reproductive decline should begin earliest in species with the longest periods of infant dependency. Data on the lions and baboons are roughly consistent with this notion: lion cubs suffer extensive mortality if they are orphaned before the age of one year and the median life expectancy of a 14-year-old female is only 1.8 years. Baboons suffer excess mortality if they are orphaned any time before two years, and the life expectancy of a 21-year-old baboon is 5.0 years.

Can this pattern account for the timing of menopause in our own species? Reproductive decline in women is pronounced by the age of 40, and data from several non-technological societies shows that 40 year-old women have an average life expectancy of approximately 18–25 years (Hill and Hurtado 1991). This is precisely the timing that would be predicted by extrapolation from the lion and baboon data if the period of human infant dependency is 10 years (Fig. 6).

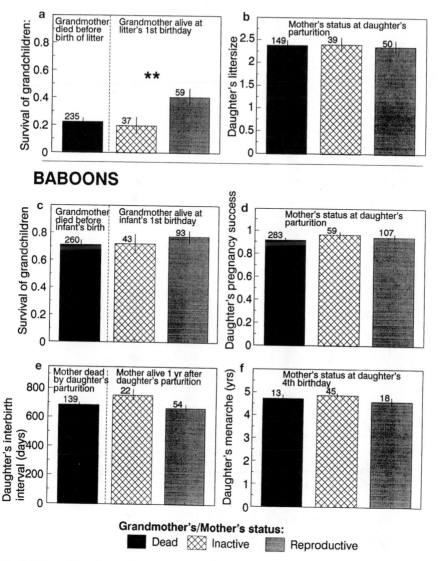

Fig. 3. Effects of female survival and reproduction on descendants' productivity. Females were "inactive" if they had not reproduced during the prior year and for six months thereafter; otherwise they were "reproductive." For lions: a, Proportion of grandchildren in each litter that survived to one year (** = p < 0.01). b, Daughters' average littersize. For baboons: c, Proportion of infant grandchildren that survived to one year. d, Proportion of daughters' pregnancies that reached full term. e, Interval from birth of surviving grandchild until the next live birth. f, Age at which daughters reached menarche. The only significant effect was in lions, where grandchildren of reproductively active grandmothers enjoyed higher survival

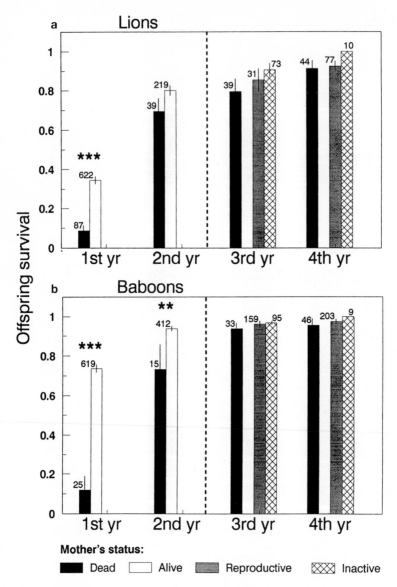

Fig. 4. Effects of female survival and subsequent reproduction on offspring survival in a, lions and b, baboons. Survival was significantly lower for animals orphaned during their first year in both species and during the second year in baboons. The typical interbirth interval for both species is two years (represented by the vertical lines), so effects of subsequent reproduction could only be measured in older juveniles. Mothers who gave birth before their prior offspring's second birthday were "reproductive" for the juvenile's third year, otherwise they were "inactive." Juvenile survival was not influenced by the mothers' reproduction. (** = p < 0.001; ** = p < 0.000)

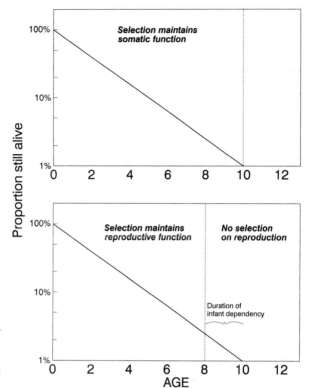

Fig. 5. Idealized survival curves for a hypothetical species with constant mortality such that only 1 % of individuals survive to the age of 10 years. The duration of infant dependency is two years

Discussions of the human menopause often confound the *existence* of menopause with the *timing* of menopause. Reproductive cessation is a fundamental feature of mammalian females; any hominid ancestor who lived long enough would have experienced reproductive senescence. Thus, models of adaptive menopause should not center on *whether* women undergo reproductive cessation but *when*. Humans show prolonged periods of infant dependency, but is the effect of being orphaned at 10 years of age really strong enough to account for a midlife menopause as we have plotted in Figure 6? Are we even correct in assuming that human menopause occurs in the middle of the life span? The survival curves of contemporary non-industrial societies may bear little resemblance to life in a pre-technological world. We have no idea what percentage of stone-age 40-year-olds ever experienced menopause – let alone reached 58–65 years of age.

Regardless of the precise demography of our ancestors, women certainly differ from most other mammalian females in their relatively rapid reproductive rates. A woman's interbirth interval is far shorter than the duration of infant dependency, thus she may often have to divide her care among an age-graded brood of offspring. If parturition becomes sufficiently hazardous with increasing maternal age, menopause could theoretically improve a woman's lifetime fitness

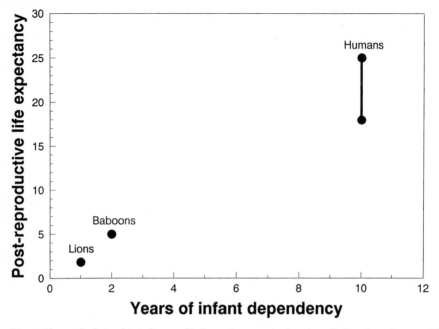

Fig. 6. Observed relationship in lions and baboons between the duration of infant dependency and the median life expectancy at the onset of reproductive decline. Values for humans assume a 10-year period of infant dependency and are extrapolated as follows: for baboons (life expectancy at the onset of reproductive decline)/ (duration of infant dependency) = 5.0 years/2 years = 2.5; for lions, 1.8 years/ 1 year = 1.8

(Williams 1957; Rogers 1993). However, if this idea is correct, women always undergo menopause before reaching the presumed age of high-risk childbirth, and thus the risks of late-aged pregnancy cannot be measured. How can this hypothesis ever be tested?

Menopause results from the loss of ovarian function (Wise et al. 1996); the success of in vitro fertilization depends on the age of the donor rather than of the recipient (Stolwijk et al. 1997). Post-menopausal women can be impregnated artificially, and this procedure provides an experimental population in their 50s and 60s. Although these are wealthy women with access to the most advanced forms of obstetrical care, any measure of their health during pregnancy would be very valuable.

It should be noted, however, that the "risk of pregnancy" hypothesis ultimately depends on patterns of senescence: aging women are presumed to be increasingly vulnerable to the rigors of childbirth. Thus any "advantages" of menopause would merely reinforce the pattern of reproductive senescence illustrated by Fig. 5. Indeed, newspaper accounts of post-menopausal pregnancies largely focussed on whether these women would be able to cope with the rigors of raising teenaged children.

The "grannie effect" might also accelerate the human menopause: if women typically reach middle age soon after their firstborn offspring have started producing grandchildren, the grandmother might leave more descendants if she helped her adult children rather than tried to continue breeding herself. In its most extreme form, this argument has been proposed as the sole explanation for menopause, but it is difficult to accept on at least two grounds.

First, most helping behavior is facultative in social vertebrates: yearling birds generally remain as "helpers at the nest" only when they lack breeding opportunities themselves (see Stacey and Koenig 1990). Why should women be "hardwired" to stop reproduction when they may reach middle age without any adult offspring? In fact, menopause occurs at significantly younger ages in women who have never had children (van Noord et al. 1997). A grannie-related menopause should show precisely the opposite pattern.

Second, in many social species, adults coerce their offspring into acting as helpers. In several carnivores and non-human primates, the social unit consists of an adult breeding pair and their mature offspring. If there is reproductive suppression within the group, the dominant pair always suppresses the subordinates. Why would middle-aged matriarchs forego their own breeding opportunities in favor of their sons and daughters? According to kinship theory, a matriarch would have to raise an additional two grandchildren for every child she "lost" through an early menopause.

The "grannie hypothesis" is most plausible if we again assume some underlying level of senescence. As aging women become less able to raise their own offspring, they might eventually reach a point where they are better off directing their remaining energies toward grandchildren. This idea is presented graphically in Figure 7. A woman's own reproductive rate is assumed to decline after the age of 40, whereas there is a more gradual decline in the number of *additional* surviving grandchildren that would be produced through intensive grandmaternal care. Although a woman might never enhance her children's reproduction sufficiently to overcome the costs of menopause during her prime years, her personal rate of reproduction might eventually decline below her impact on the production of grandchildren – at which point menopause would finally be favored.

Thus if a "grannie effect" were particularly important in human evolution, we might expect women to show a more precipitous decline in reproductive performance than females in other species (with the onset of reproductive decline still being set by the duration of infant dependency, as in Fig. 5). However, the rate of decline in human reproduction is very similar to patterns in lions and baboons (Fig. 1 b,d), suggesting that the human menopause may not be that different from other species after all.

A more rigorous test of this idea could be performed by tracking women's competence as mothers and as grandmothers through their 30s and 40s to see if maternal competency decreases more rapidly than their proficiency as grandmothers (as assumed in Fig. 7). But the key test (as we performed in Fig. 3) will be to determine whether women are ineffective grandmothers when they are trying to raise their own infants. Unless there is a trade-off between maternal care and grandmaternal care, there would be no reason for women to stop reproduction.

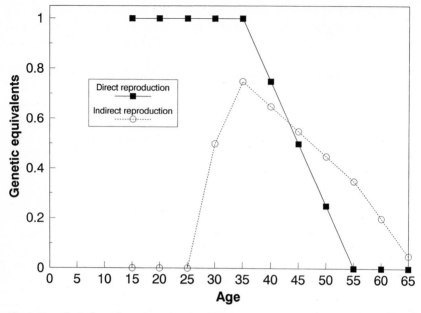

Fig. 7. Hypothetical age changes in a female's ability to produce surviving offspring ("direct reproduction") or surviving grandchildren ("indirect reproduction"). Units of "genetic equivalents" are arbitrary, but a female must help her sons and/or daughters raise an additional two grandchildren to have the same genetic equivalent as one offspring of her own. Maternal productivity is assumed to decline at a constant rate from the age of 40. A female's capacity for indirect reproduction depends on the maturation of her firstborn offspring and then declines with advancing age. As drawn here, indirect reproduction exceeds direct reproduction at 45 years

Does any of this matter? Unlike the most extreme rendering of the reproductive senescence hypothesis, our view suggests that women are adapted to survive menopause – but not for long. To many modern women, menopause is an unremitting biological clock that limits the age at which they can start a family. For women who started their families much earlier, reproductive senescence may enforce a more exclusive interest in grandchildren, but as one of my friends in her 50s once put it to me, "The great thing about grandchildren is that their parents take them home when you get tired!"

References

Altmann SA (1970) The pregnancy sign in savannah baboons. Lab Anim Digest 6:7–10

Angier N (1999) Woman: an intimate geography. New York, Houghton-Mifflen

Charlesworth B (1980) Evolution in age-structured populations. Cambridge, Cambridge University Press

Finch CE (1990) Longevity, senescence and the genome. Chicago, University of Chicago Press

Gouzoules S, Gouzoules H (1987) In: Smuts BB et al. (eds) Primate Societies. Chicago, University of Chicago Press, 299–305

Hamilton WD (1966) The moulding of senescence by natural selection. J Theoret Biol 12:12–45

Hawkes K, O'Connell JF, Blurton-Jones N (1997) Hadza women's time allocation, offspring provisioning, and the evolution of long postmenopausal life spans. Curr Anthropol 38:551–565

Hill K, Hurtado AM (1991) The evolution of premature reproductive senescence and menopause in human females: an evaluation of the "Grandmother Hypothesis." Human Nature 2:313–350

Lauerman WC, Platenberg RC, Cain JE, Deeney VFX (1992) Age-related disk degeneration: Preliminary report of a naturally occurring baboon model. J Spinal Disord 5:170–174

Ledford FF (1998) Report to the Southwestern Foundation for Biomedical Research

Nesse RM, Williams GC (1994) Why we get sick. New York, Random House

Packer C, Pusey AE (1997) Divided we fall: cooperation among lions. Sci Amer 276:52–59

Packer C, Tatar M, Collins DA (1998) Reproductive cessation in female mammals. Nature 392:807–811

Pusey AE, Packer C (1994) Non-offspring nursing in social carnivores: minimizing the costs. Behav Ecol 5:362–374

Rogers AR (1993) Why menopause? Evol Ecol 7:406–420

Sapolsky RM, Finch CE (1999) The Alzheimer's lottery. Nat Hist 108(9):22–29

Sherman PW (1998) The evolution of menopause. Nature 392:759–761

Stacey PB, Koenig WD (1990) Cooperative breeding in birds. Cambridge, Cambridge University Press

Stolwijk AM, Zielhuis GA, Sauer MV, Hamilton CJCM, Paulson RJ (1997) The impact of the woman's age on the success of standard and donor in vitro fertilization. Fertil Steril 67:702–710

van Noord PAH, Dubas JS, Dorland M, Boersma H, te Velde E (1997) Age at natural menopause in a population-based screening cohort: the role of menarche, fecundity, and lifestyle factors. Fertil Steril 68:95–102

vom Saal FS, Finch CE, Nelson JF (1994) In: Knobil E, Neill JD (eds) The physiology of reproduction. Second Edition. New York, Raven Press, 1213–1314

Williams GC (1957) Pleiotropy, natural selection, and the evolution of senescence. Evolution 11:398–411

Wise PM, Krajnak KM, Kashon ML (1996) Menopause: The aging of multiple pacemakers. Science 273:67–70

Androgen Deficiency in Aging Males and Healthy Aging

J. E. Morley

As life span has increased, it has become more important to focus on the needs of humans in the second half of their lives. In women this has led to increased enthusiasm for estrogen replacement, not only to treat menopausal symptoms but also to prevent bone loss and perhaps to delay the onset of cardiovascular disease and Alzheimer's disease. The trade-off of these potential benefits has been the role of estrogens in promoting endometrial carcinoma and perhaps breast cancer. Despite the large enthusiasm for hormonal replacement in women, there has been much less enthusiasm for exploring the potential benefits for hormonal replacement in men.

While men die younger than women, they tend on the whole to have better function at any given age. In addition, the mortality differential between men and women in Europe and North America has led to the assumption that the male hormone, testosterone, in some way is responsible for the earlier mortality

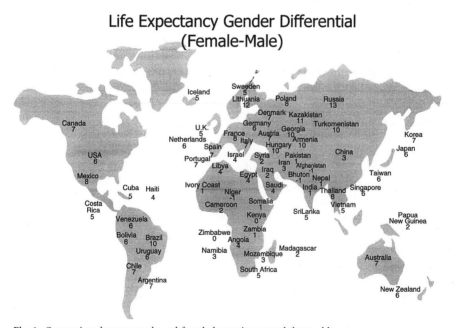

Fig. 1. Comparison between male and female longevity around the world

Robine et al. (Eds.)
Sex and Longevity: Sexuality, Gender,
Reproduction, Parenthood
© Springer-Verlag Berlin Heidelberg 2000

in males. However, there is evidence that the longevity differential between men and women is a European phenomenon (Fig. 1). As can be seen, in parts of the Asian subcontinent men live longer than women, and in the subcontinent and in Central Africa the longevity differential is much less marked. In addition, Seventh Day Adventists and the Amish fail to show the female longevity advantage. These findings suggest that the female longevity advantage, when it is seen, is not due to testosterone but to some other environmental or genetic factor.

There are a series of clear declines in physiological function with aging in males. These declines include age-related cognitive function, vision and hearing, anorexia, hypodipsia, muscle mass and strength, maximal voluntary oxygen consumption, bone density, libido and sexual function. Recent findings have suggested that testosterone declines in parallel with these physiological changes. This raises the questions of whether or not the age-related testosterone is involved in the pathogenesis of some of these changes and if so whether testosterone treatment would reverse some of these changes? A third question is whether or not testosterone replacement therapy can reverse some of these age-related changes? This chapter will address each of these questions.

The Effect of Aging on Testosterone

There are now numerous cross-sectional studies that have demonstrated a decline in testosterone with aging (Morley and Perry 1999; Gray et al. 1991). This finding has recently been confirmed in a longitudinal study (Morley et al. 1997a; Fig. 2). Controversy exists concerning the appropriate measurement for testosterone. With aging, there is an increase in sex hormone binding globulin. This spuriously increases the total testosterone level in aging males. The tissue available (bioavailable) testosterone consists of both the free testosterone and that which is bound to albumin. Most workers in the field feel that this is the most appropriate measurement of testosterone status, though the testosterone glucuronide measurement has also been suggested. Recently Vermeulen and colleagues (1999) provided evidence that a free testosterone index (which takes into account the binding capacity of sex hormone binding globulin) may be a useful proxy. Neither the free androgen index (testosterone divided by sex hormone binding globulin) nor the free testosterone analog assays should be used in older persons.

The reason for the decline in testosterone with aging is multifactorial. With aging there is a decline in the ability of the Leydig cells to produce testosterone in response to gonadotrophins (Harman et al. 1980). However, unlike the situation in female menopause where loss of sex hormone production results in an elevation of luteinizing hormone (LH), in males LH does not increase in concert with the fall in LH. This finding suggests a failure in the hypothalamic pituitary unit with aging. Decreased responsiveness of the pituitary to gonadotrophin-releasing hormone was confirmed by Korenman and his colleagues (1990).

However, the major change with aging appears to be the failure of the hypothalamus to maintain appropriate pulsatile secretion of the hypothalamic-

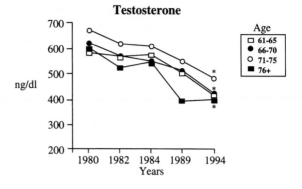

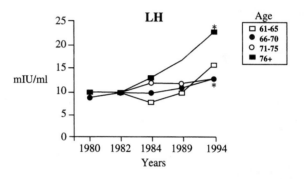

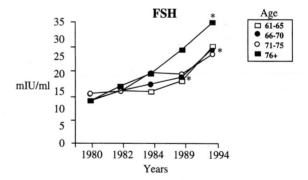

Fig. 2. Longitudinal changes in testosterone, luteinizing hormone (LH) and follicle-stimulating hormone (FSH) in older males. (From Morley et al. 1997)

* $p < 0.01$ different from 1980 value

pituitary-gonadal axis. In healthy aging there is a decline in the amplitude of LH release associated with an increase in secretory events (Mulligan et al. 1998). This is associated with a more irregular LH secretion (Pincus et al. 1996). Veldhuis and his colleagues (1999) have suggested that these changes in LH secretion represent a part of a more extensive disorganization of the hypothalamic-neural network, with aging that results not only in progressive reproductive failure but also other nonreproductiive biological feedback-control systems. These findings pos-

tulate an important role for a central nervous system biological clock in the pathophysiology of the aging process.

An overview of the changes in the hypothalamic-pituitary-gonadal axis with
aging is given in Figure 3.

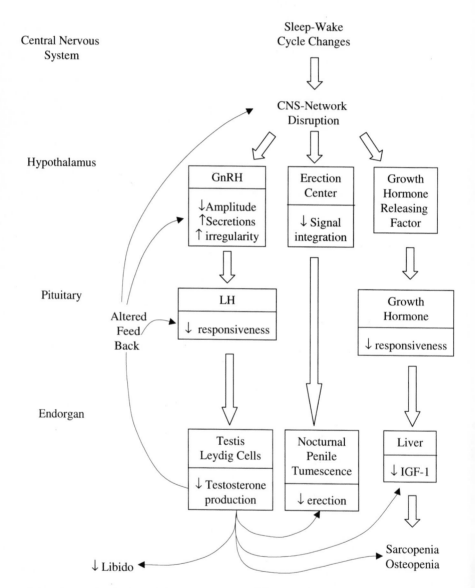

Fig. 3. Changes in the hypothalamic-pituitary-gonadal axis with aging. GnRH, gonadotrophin-
releasing hormone; IGF-I, insulin-like growth factor; CNS, Central Nervous System

Historical Development of the Concept of Male Menopause

The concept that the testes played a role in male libido and strength was well established by Galen and Rleny. In addition, over 2000 years ago Ayurvedic medicine suggested that ingestion of testes would cure impotence.

The concept that the decline in testosterone with aging is responsible for aging changes in strength and behavior was first popularized by Brown-Sequard in 1889. He suggested that self-injection of testosterone extracts resulted in improved strength and prevented him from falling asleep after dinner! While the medical establishment rejected his findings, as shown by a derogatory editorial in the British Medical Journal in 1890 entitled the "Pentacle of Rejuvenescence," others embraced his findings and the utilization of injections of testicular extracts was embraced by many such older persons. This led in the 1920s to the chimpanzee testicular transplantation craze that was first popularized by Serge Voronof in Europe (Hamilton 1986).

After the isolation and synthesis of testosterone in the 1930s, in 1940 Thomas and Hill were the first to report the successful treatment of the male climacteric with testosterone propionate. In 1944, Heller and Myers reported an improvement in male climacteric symptoms with testosterone compared to sesame oil as placebo.

Testosterone and Sexuality

Numerous studies have demonstrated that testosterone deficiency is associated with decline in libido and that testosterone replacement reverses this phenomenon. Schiavi and his colleagues (1991) demonstrated strong correlations in older males between bioavailable testosterone and frequency of sexual thoughts, frequency of desire for sex and easiness of becoming aroused. Both Hajjar et al. (1997) and Morales et al. (1997) demonstrated improvement in libido in older men receiving testosterone replacement. In younger hypogonadal males a synthetic anabolic testosterone that is not converted to dihydrotestosterone has been shown to have similar effects on libido, demonstrating that dihydrotestosterone is not responsible for these effects.

The effects of testosterone on erectile function is less clear. Billington and his colleagues (1981) showed that testosterone increased nocturnal penile tumescence response in older hypogonadal males when compared to placebo. Testosterone is necessary for nitric oxide synthase (NOS) activity. NOS elaborates nitric oxide, which in turn causes smooth muscle relaxation and penile tumescence. More studies are needed in this area.

Sarcopenia and the Age Related Decline in Male Hormones

Sarcopenia ("fading of the flesh") is defined as a progressive decrease in skeletal muscle mass and strength. Sarcopenia is believed to be a major factor in the pathophysiology of age-related decline in function and the increased propensity to have injurious falls. The causes of sarcopenia are multifactorial (Fig 4). However, it would appear that the decline in testosterone with aging may be a pivotal trigger in the pathogenesis of testosterone.

Baumgartner et al. (1999) demonstrated that in older males the major factors predicting a decline in muscle mass and strength are free testosterone, insulin-like growth factor 1 and physical activity. In our study of inner city older African Americans, we have demonstrated a similar relationship between bioavailable testosterone and strength and functional status (unpublished studies).

Testosterone has been demonstrated to increase strength and muscle mass and decrease fat mass in both healthy young and hypogonadal males (Bross et al. 1999). In general, these authors have shown an increase in muscle strength and in free fat mass and a decrease in body fat (Table 1). It is important to realize that these studies have been limited in the numbers treated and that inclusion criteria have been variable. The majority utilized testosterone injections, which produced supraphysiological doses. One study entered a large number of men who were not hypogonadal and required questionable analytic techniques to demonstrate effects (Snyder et al. 1999a).

Of the six studies, three lasted for three months or less and only one was placebo controlled. One study lasted for one year and two studies for three years; all

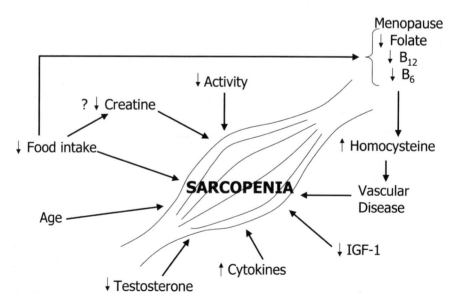

Fig. 4. The causes of sarcopenia

Table 1. Effects of testosterone replacement in older males

Study	Age (years)	Treatment	Duration	Free fat mass	Muscle strength
Tenover (1992)	60–75	Injection	3 months	Increase	None
Morley et al. (1993)	60–89	Injection	3 months	No change	Increase
Urban et al. (1995)	67±2	Injection	4 weeks	Not done	Increase
Sih et al. (1997)	51–79	Injection	12 months	No change	Increase
Snyder et al. (1999)	73±0.8	Scrotal patch	36 months	Increase	None
Tenover (1998)	60+	Injection	36 months	Increase	Increase

were placebo controlled. The second study by Tenover (1998) has not been published in detail. A seventh study by the Johns Hopkins Group appears to have similar findings but has not yet been published in any form.

At present, while testosterone therapy appears to improve muscle function, there is no data to confirm which older subjects are most amenable to testosterone treatment and what, the optimal dose is. In addition, the optimal duration of therapy and the effect of testosterone withdrawal are unknown.

Leptin and Fat Mass

Leptin is a peptide hormone produced from adipose tissue. In animals its major effects are to decrease food intake, increase resting metabolic rate and regulate the release of LH. Circulating levels of leptin correlate well with total fat mass. Females have higher leptin levels than males even after correction for fat mass, suggesting that sex hormones may play a role in the regulation of leptin secretion.

Baumgartner and his colleagues (1999) have demonstrated that, while leptin levels fall in females beyond 60 years of age in concert with the decline in fat mass, levels increase in males. Multivariant analysis suggested that the increase was due to the fall in testosterone. These findings for males were seen not only cross-sectionally but also longitudinally. In their testosterone replacement study in older hypogonadal men, Sih et al. (1997) demonstrated that testosterone decreased leptin levels.

Osteoporosis

As in females, bone mineral density declines with age in males. In young males hypogonadism results in a lower peak bone mass and a failure to maintain bone mass following puberty. Whether the changes in bone mass are directly related to testosterone or secondary to aromatization to estrogen is controversial. A man with estrogen resistance has been reported to have low bone mineral density (Smith et al. 1994).

With aging, males have an increase in hip fractures. These hip fractures are associated with a higher mortality than that seen in women. In older males hypogonadism is strongly associated with vertebral crush fractures (Baillie et al. 1992) and with minimal trauma hip fracture (Stanley et al. 1991; Jackson et al. 1992). Despite this, it has been extraordinarily difficult to demonstrate an association between the fall in bone mineral density and the decline in serum testosterone in older males (Meier et al. 1987; Murphy et al. 1993; Rudman et al. 1994; Drinka et al. 1993). Recently some studies have suggested that estrogen levels are better associated with bone mineral density than are testosterone levels (Greendale et al. 1997; Khosla et al. 1998; Slemenda et al. 1997). Utilizing a casual modeling technique Center and her colleagues (1999) suggested that low estradiol, high sex hormone binding globulin, low free testosterone and high parathyroid hormone together accounted for approximately 5% of the loss of bone mineral density at the femoral neck. Estradiol appeared to be a more important predictor of bone mineral density than did free testosterone.

Reid et al. (1996) reported improvement in bone mineral density in middle aged males receiving steroids who were treated with testosterone. Snyder et al. (1999b) found that testosterone increased bone mineral density in older males who had very low serum testosterone levels. Tenover (1998) found marked increases in lumbar and femoral bone mineral density in older males. In her study blocking conversion to dihydrotestosterone did not inhibit the increases in bone mineral density. As testosterone is aromatized to estradiol, these findings do not settle the controversy of whether the effects are due to testosterone per se or secondary to the conversion of testosterone to estradiol.

Cognitive Function

Cognitive function declines with age in males (Barrett-Connor et al. 1999). In epidemiological studies, bioavailable testosterone has been demonstrated to correlate with this decline in cognitive function in older males (Morley et al. 1997b; Barrett-Connor et al. 1999). In younger males a number of studies have suggested that the relationship between testosterone and spatial cognition shows a quadratic (U-shaped) relationship (Moffat and Hampson 1996; Gouchie and Kimura 1991; McKeever and Deyo 1990).

Three studies in older males have examined the effects of testosterone replacement on cognitive function. Two (Janowsky et al. 1994; Herbst et al. 1999) showed improvement in visuospatial cognitive performance. Using a wider assay of cognitive tests Sih et al. (1997) failed to demonstrate an improvement in cognition.

The Samp8 Mouse; Testosterone and Alzheimer's Disease

The SAMP8 mouse spontaneously overproduces amyloid-β protein and presenilin 1 (Flood and Morley 1998). This overproduction is associated with early onset of deficits in acquisition and retention compared to other mice. We have previously demonstrated that amyloid-β-protein produces retention deficits in mice (Flood et al. 1994). In the SAMP8 mouse we demonstrated that antibodies to amyloid-β-protein or antisense oligonucleotides to amyloid precursor protein will reverse the acquisition and retention deficits in these mice. Amyloid plaques occur in these mice, but only some months after the onset of cognitive deficits.

A number of studies have suggested that estrogen may be protective against of Alzheimer's disease (Birge 1996). We have found that the SAMP8 mice have a rapid decline in testosterone levels in parallel with the decline in cognitive function (Flood et al. 1995). Testosterone replacement in these mice reverses the acquisition and retention deficits. Testosterone treatment results in a marked decrease in amyloid precursor protein in the hippocampus and in the amygdala. These findings strongly suggest a possible role for testosterone in the treatment of Alzheimer's disease.

Cardiovascular Disease

Contrary to popular opinion, low testosterone levels have been demonstrated to be associated with atherosclerotic cardiovascular disease (Barrett-Connor 1995). Animal studies have shown that testosterone produces coronary artery vasodilation through the release of nitric oxide (Yue et al. 1995). Testosterone treatment reverses ST depression both acutely (Rosano et al. 1999; Webb et al. 1999) and chronically (Jaffe 1977). A retrospective study demonstrated no increase in cardiovascular disease during testosterone treatment (Hajjar et al. 1997). Overall, these studies suggest that testosterone may be protective against atherosclerotic coronary artery disease.

Prostate Disease

While there is much belief that testosterone is important in the pathogenesis of prostate disease, there is surprisingly little evidence to support this concept. Recently evidence has emerged that estradiol may be more important than testosterone in promoting prostate growth. Lobund-Wistar rats treated with dihydrotestosterone developed less adenocarcinoma than did placebo controls (Pollard 1998). Small increases in prostatic specific antigen (PSA) occur when hypogonadal males are first treated, but PSA levels tend to remain in the normal range. Retrospective studies have not found any increase in prostate disease in older males receiving testosterone (Hajjar et al. 1997).

Hemoglobin

With aging, there is a 1–2 g/dl fall in hemoglobin levels. Testosterone treatment increases hemoglobin levels. This effect of testosterone does not involve erythropoetin, but rather appears to be a direct effect on the bone marrow has an indirect effect by increasing insulin growth factor-1.

Adam Questionnaire

St. Louis University has developed an Androgen Deficiency in Aging Males (ADAM) questionnaire to detect symptoms of testosterone deficiency in older males (Tab. 2). This questionnaire has been shown to have high sensitivity and adequate specificity. Testosterone treatment in males reverses many of these symptoms. The most common cause of a false positive is depression.

Conclusion

Tissue available levels of testosterone decline steadily with aging, resulting in many older males being hypogonadal. In addition, rodent studies have suggested that aging may be associated with a decrease in androgen receptors (Haji et al. 1980). There are now a number of studies supporting the use of testosterone replacement therapy for the reversal of age-related sarcopenia, osteoporosis and cognitive dysfunction. The effects of long-term administration of testosterone on longevity remain to be determined. At present it would appear prudent to offer testosterone replacement therapy to older males who have symptoms and whose bioavailable testosterone levels fall below those of the range for normal young men. However, it is useful to remember the Greek myth of Daedelus and Icarus. To escape from Crete, Daedelus fashioned wax wings for himself and Icarus. He warned Icarus not to fly too close to the sun. Unfortunately, Icarus failed to heed this warning and plummeted to his death in the Mediterranean. Similar caution

Table 2. ADAM questionnaire[a]

1. Do you have a decrease in libido (sex drive)?
2. Do you have a lack of energy?
3. Do you have a decrease in strength and/or endurance?
4. Have you lost height?
5. Have you noticed a decreased "enjoyment of life"?
6. Are you sad and/or grumpy?
7. Are your erections less strong?
8. Have you noted a recent deterioration in your ability to play sports?
9. Are you falling asleep after dinner?
10. Has there been a recent deterioration in your work performance?

[a] Positive answers to 1, 7 or any three others suggest hypogonadism

should be kept in mind as we probe the risk/benefit ratio of hormonal replacement therapy in older males. An important question will be whether low or high dose testosterone is the appropriate replacement therapy. In addition, the possible role of selective androgen receptor molecules needs to be determined.

References

Baillie SP, Davison CE, Johnson FJ, Francis RM (1992) Pathogenesis of vertebral crush fractures in men. Age Ageing 21:139–141

Barrett-Connor EL (1995) Testosterone and risk factors for cardiovascular disease in men. Diabet Metab 21:156–161

Barrett-Connor E, Goodman-Gruen D, Patay B (1999) Endogenous sex hormones and cognitive function in older men. J Clin Endocrinol Metab 84(10):3681–3685

Baumgartner RN, Waters DL, Morley JE, Patrick P, Montoya GD, Garry PJ (1999) Age-related changes in sex hormones affect the sex difference in serum leptin independent of changes in body fat. Metabolism 48:378–384

Billington CJ, Mooradian AD, Duff L, Lange P, Morley JE (1991) Testosterone therapy in impotent patients with normal testosterone. Clin Res 31:718A

Birge SJ (1996) Is there a role for estrogen replacement therapy in the prevention and treatment of dementia? J Am Geriatr Soc 44(7):865–70

Bross R, Javanbakht M, Bhasin S (1999) Anabolic interventions for aging-associated sarcopenia. J Clin Endocrinol Metab 84(10):3420–3430

Brown-Sequard CE (1889) The physiological and therapeutic of animal testicular extract based on several experiments in man. Physiol Norm Pathol 115:739–746

Center JR, Nguyen TV, Sambrook PN, Eisman JA (1999) Hormonal and biochemical parameters in the determination of osteoporosis in elderly men. J Clin Endocrinol Metab 84(10):3626–3635

Cherrier M, Craft S, Plymate S, Brammer J (1998) Effects of testosterone on cognition in healthy older men. Endocrin Abstr 98:2–643

Drinka PJ, Olson J, Bauwens S, Voetzs SK, Carlson I, Wilson M (1993) Lack of association between free testosterone and bone density separate from age in elderly males. Calcif Tissue Int 52:67–69

Flood JF, Morley JE, Roberts E (1994) An amyloid beta-protein fragment, A beta[12–28], equipotently impairs post-training memory processing when injected into different limbic system structures. Brain Res 663(2):271–6

Flood JF, Morley JE (1998) Learning and memory in the SAMP8 mouse. Neurosci Biobehav Rev 22:1–20

Flood JF, Farr SA, Kaiser FE, La Regina M, Morley JE (1995) Age-related decrease of plasma testosterone in SAMP8 mice: Replacement improves age-related impairment of learning and memory. Physiol Behav 57:669–673

Gouchie C, Kimura D (1991) The relationship between testosterone levels and cognitive ability patterns. Psychoneuroendocrinology 16:323–334

Gray A, Berlin JA, McKinlay JB, Longcope C (1991) An examination of research design effects on the association of testosterone and male aging: Results of a meta-analysis. J Clin Epidemiol 44:671–684

Greendale GA, Edelstein S, Barrett-Connor E (1997) Endogenous sex steroids and bone mineral density in older women and men: the Rancho Bernardo Study. J Bone Miner Res 12:1833–1843

Haji M, Kato KI, Nawata H, Ibayashi H (1980) Age-related changes in the concentrations of cytosol receptors for sex steroid hormones in the hypothalamus and pituitary gland of the rat. Brain Res. 204(2):373–86

Hajjar RR, Kaiser FE, Morley JE (1997) Outcomes of long-term testosterone replacement in older hypogonadal males: A retrospective analysis. J Clin Endocrinol Metab 82:3793–3796

Hamilton D (1986) The monkey gland affair. New York, Chatto & Windus

Harman SM, Tsitouras PD (1980) Reproductive hormones in aging men: I. Measurement of sex steroids, basal luteinizing hormone, and Leydig cell response to human chorionic gonadotropin. J Clin Endocrinol Metab 51:35–40

Heller CG, Myers GB (1944) The male climacteric: Its symptomatology, diagnosis and treatment. JAMA 126:472–477

Herbst KL, Anawalt BD, Chernier M, Craft S, Matsumoto AM, Bremner WJ (1999) Testosterone administration improves spatial memory in normal men. Proc 81st Meeting Endocrine Soc P3-363

Jackson JA, Riggs MW, Spiekerman AM (1992) Testosterone deficiency as a risk factor for hip fractures in men: a case-control study. Am J Med Sci 304:4–8

Jaffe MD (1977) Effect of testosterone cypionate on postexercise ST segment depression. Brit Heart J 39:1217–1222

Janowsky JS, Oviatt SK, Orwoll ES (1994) Testosterone influences spatial cognition in older men. Behav Neurosci 108:325–332

Khosla S, Melton L, Atkinson EJ, O'Fallon WM, Klee GG, Riggs BL (1998) Relationship of serum sex steroid levels and bone turnover markers with bone mineral density in men and women: a key role for bioavailable estrogen. J Clin Endocrinol Metab 83:2266–74

Korenman SG, Morley JE, Mooradian AD, Davis SS, Kaiser FE, Silver AJ, Viosca S, Gazza D (1990) Secondary hypogonadism in older men: its relation to impotence. J Clin Endocrinol Metab 71:963–969

McKeever WF, Deyo RA (1990) Testosterone, dihydrotestosterone and spatial task performance of males. Bull Psychosom Soc 28:305–308

Meier DE, Orwoll ES, Keenan EJ, Fagerstrom RM (1987) Marked decline in trabecular bone mineral content in healthy men with age: lack of association with sex steroid levels. J Am Geriatr Soc 35:189–197

Moffat SD, Hampson E (1996) A curvilinear relationship between testosterone and spatial cognition in humans: possible influence of hand preference. Psychoneuroendocrinology 21:323–337

Morales A, Johnston B, Heaton JP, Lundie M (1997) Testosterone supplementation for hypogonadal impotence: Assessment of biochemical measures and therapeutic outcomes. J Urol 157:849–854

Morley JE and Perry HM III (1999) Androgen deficiency in aging men. Med Clin N Am 83(5):1279

Morley JE, Kaiser FE, Perry HM 3rd, Patrick P, Morley PM, Stauber PM, Vellas B, Baumgartner RN, Garry PJ (1997a) Longitudinal changes in testosterone, luteinizing hormone, and follicle-stimulating hormone in healthy older men. Metabolism 46:410–413

Morley JE, Kaiser F, Raum WJ, Perry HM 3rd, Flood JF, Jensen J, Silver A, Roberts E (1997b) Potentially predictive and manipulable blood serum correlates of aging in the healthy human male: Progressive decreases in bioavailable testosterone, dehydroepiandrosterone sulfate, and the ratio of insulin-like growth factor-1 to growth hormone. Proc Natl Acad Sci USA 94:7537–42

Morley JE, Perry HM 3rd, Kaiser FE, Kraenzle D, Jensen J, Houston K, Mattammal M, Perry HM Jr (1993) Effects of testosterone replacement therapy in old hypogonadal males: A preliminary study. J Am Geriatr Soc 41:149–152

Mulligan T, Iranmanesh A, Johnson ML, Straume M, Veldhuis JD (1997) Aging alters feed-forward and feedback linkages between LH and testosterone in healthy men. Am J Physiol 273(r):R1407–13

Murphy S, Khaw K, Cassidy A, Compston JE (1993) Sex hormones and bone mineral density in elderly men. Bone Miner 20:133–140

Pincus SM, Veldhuis JD, Mulligan T, Iranmanesh A, Evans WS (1997) Effects of age on the irregularity of LH and FSH serum concentrations in women and men. Am J Physiol 273(5):E989–95

Pollard M (1998) Dihydrotestosterone prevents spontaneous adenocarcinomas in the prostate-seminal vesicle in aging L-W rats. Prostate 36:168–171

Reid IR, Wattie DJ, Evans MC, Stapleton JP (1996) Testosterone therapy in glucocorticoid-treated men. Arch Intern Med 156:1173–1177

Rosano GMC, Leonardo F, Pagnotta P, Pelliccia F, Panina G, Cerquetani E, della Monica PL, Bonfigli B, Volpe M, Chierchia SL (1999) Acute anti-ischemic effect of testosterone in men with coronary artery disease. Circulation 99(13):1666–1670

Rudman D, Drinka PJ, Wilson CR, Mattson DE, Scherman F, Cuisinier MC, Schultz S (1994) Relations of endogenous anabolic hormones and physical activity to bone mineral density and lead body mass in elderly men. Clin Endocrinol (Oxf) 40:653–661

Schiavi RC, Schreiner-Engel P, White D, Mandeli J (1991) The relationship between pituitary-gonadal function and sexual behavior in healthy aging men. Psychosom Med 53:363–374

Sih R, Morley JE, Kaiser FE, Perry HM 3rd, Patrick P, Ross C (1997) Testosterone replacement in older hypogonadal men: A 12-month randomized controlled trial. J Clin Endocrinol Metab 82:1661–1667

Slemenda CW, Longscope C, Zhou L, Hui SL, Peacock M, Johnston CC (1997) Sex steroids and bone mass in older men. J Clin Invest 100:1755–1759

Smith EP, Boyd J, Frank GR, Takahashi H, Cohen RM, Speckee B, Williams TC, Lubahn DB, Korack KS (1994) Estrogen resistance caused by a mutation in the estrogen-receptor gene in a man. New Engl J Med 331:1056–1061

Snyder PJ, Peachey H, Hannoush P, Berlin JA, Loh L, Lenrow DA, Holmes JH, Dlewati A, Santanna J, Rosen CJ, Strom BL (1999) Effect of testosterone treatment on body composition and muscle strength in men over 65 years of age. J Clin Endocrinol Metab 84(8):2647–2653

Snyder PJ, Peachey H, Hannoush P, Berlin JA, Loh L, Holmes JH, Dlewati A, Staley J, Santanna J, Kapoor SC, Attie MF, Haddad JG, Strom BL (1999) Effect of testosterone treatment on bone mineral density in men over 65 years of age. J Clin Endocrinol Metab 84(6):1966–1972

Stanley HL, Schmitt BP, Foses RM, Deiss WP (1991) Does hypogognadism contribute to the occurrence of a minimal trauma hip fracture in elderly men? J Am Geriatr Soc 39:766–771

Tenover JS (1992) Effects of testosterone supplementation in the aging male. J Clin Endocrinol Metab 75(4):1092–8

Tenover JS (1998) Androgen replacement therapy to reverse and/or prevent age-associated sarcopenia in men. Baillieres Clin Endocrinol Metab 12(3):419–425

Urban RJ, Bodenburg YH, Gilkison C, Foxworth J, Coggan AR, Wolfe RR, Ferrando A (1995) Testosterone administration to elderly men increases skeletal muscle strength and protein synthesis. Am J Physiol 269:E820–826

Veldhuis JD, Iranmanesh A, Mulligan T, Pincus SM (1999) Disruption of the young-adult synchrony between luteinizing hormone release and oscillations in follicle-stimulating hormone, prolactin, and nocturnal penile tumescence (NPT) in healthy older men. J Clin Endocrinol Metab 84(10):3498–3505

Vermeulen A, Verdonck L, Kaufman JM (1999) A critical evaluation of simple methods for the estimation of free testosterone in serum. J Clin Endocrinol Metab 84(10):3666–3672

Webb CM, Adamson DL, de Zeigler D, Collins P (1999) Effect of acute testosterone on myocardial ischemia in men with coronary artery disease. Am J Cardiol 83(3):437

Yue P, Chatterjee K, Beale C, Poole-Wilson PA, Collins P (1995) Testosterone relaxes rabbit coronary arteries and aorta. Circulation 91:1154–1160

Patterns of Childbearing and Mortality in Norwegian Women
A 20-Year Follow-Up of Women Aged 40–96 in the 1970 Norwegian Census

M. Kumle and E. Lund

Summary

In order to study the relationship between different patterns of childbearing and longevity, we have followed married women in the 1970 Norwegian census for 20 years. The analysis was restricted to women aged 40–96, married before the age of 40, and with known information about parity, covering a total of 9 116 783 person-years with 149 044 deaths from all causes. Nulliparous women had higher mortality than parous women did in all age groups. Compared with uniparous women, adjusted for age at start of follow-up, years of education, and age at first and last birth, parous women with three children had the lowest relative risk, 0.92 (95 % confidence interval: 0.90–0.94). Age at first birth had no impact on mortality. Compared to women with a last birth before the age of 25 years, the mortality was lowest in women with a last birth at age 35 years or more, with a relative risk = 0.89 (95 % confidence interval: 0.87–0.92).

We conclude that women with few children born late in the fertile period have the lowest mortality rate for the rest of their lives.

Introduction

Is there a connection between specific patterns of childbearing and longevity in human females? A search on Medline, September 1999, revealed that although there were many studies on different patterns of childbearing in relation to incidence and specific cause of mortality (e.g. hormone-related cancers and heart diseases) in human females, only a few studies world-wide focused on the total mortality in women related to different fertility patterns (Beral 1985; Green et al. 1988; Lund 1990; Westendorp and Kirkwood 1998; Promislow 1998; Perls et al. 1997; Le-Bourg et al. 1993). The first study, based on death certificates and census information from England, showed an increased risk of death among parous women compared to nulliparous, but the design of the analysis was not optimal (Beral 1985). Another English follow-up study of the 1971 census found that nulliparous women had higher mortality than parous, and that the number of children had different effects on different causes of death (Green et al. 1988). The first large-scale study that also took into account the age of the mother at each birth in relation to total mortality was published in 1990, based on married

Robine et al. (Eds.)
Sex and Longevity: Sexuality, Gender, Reproduction, Parenthood
© Springer-Verlag Berlin Heidelberg 2000

women who participated in the 1970 Norwegian census with follow-up to 1985 (Lund 1990). The main conclusion was that postponed childbearing reduced the mortality rate.

In the late 1990s, there was renewed interest in the relationship between reproduction and longevity, based on the hypothesis that human longevity had a reproductive cost (Westendorp and Kirkwood 1998; Promislow 1998; Perls et al. 1997).

In this paper, we present a re-analysis of fertility and longevity in the Norwegian census cohort with an extended follow-up time.

Material and Methods

The 1970 Norwegian census (Vassenden 1987) included all the inhabitants of the country based on information from the National Population Register from Statistics Norway. The National Population Register is a main source of administrative information, largely because of the unique 11 digit identification number given to all persons alive at the census in 1960, and to those who were born or immigrated later. The identification number consists of date of birth, gender, and control numbers. The National Population Register is computerised and regularly updated with information on migration, immigration, emigration, and death. The pre-printed census questionnaires containing identification number, name, address, and marital status were sent to each local population registration office. The census officials visited every household to deliver the questionnaire. The informants had to correct any errors in the pre-printed information. Shortly after the census date, November 1, 1970, the questionnaires were collected by the census officials and returned to Statistics Norway.

Follow-up on mortality was obtained by a linkage based on the unique national identification number in the files of the census with that in all deaths registered by Statistics Norway in the period from November 1, 1970 to December 31, 1989. Information on emigration was obtained by linking census information with emigration reports to the National Population Register up to December 31, 1989. Individuals were excluded from the estimation of follow-up from the moment of emigration, and those who re-immigrated were included until death or until counted on December 31, 1989. Mortality rates were based on the exact person-year of follow-up computed for each woman.

Altogether 1 338 716 women, aged 20–96, in 1970 participated in the Norwegian census, representing 23 099 316 years of follow-up and 372 310 deaths in the period 1970–1989. The questions on parity were only put to women who were married at that time (Dyrvik 1976). The married women were asked about their age at marriage, number of children in the present marriage, and the age of each child (stillborn not included). Because of the lack of parity information, widows, divorced women and unmarried women were excluded from the main analyses. Women aged 20–39 were excluded since they might give birth to children after 1970. Women aged 40 years or more had almost finished their fertility history, and added less than 0.1 children on average to the 1970 figures (Brunborg 1988). All the women were asked about their own level of education, primary school (seven years), or higher education (eight years or more).

These main analyses were restricted to women aged 40–96, married before the age of 40 and with known parity, totalling 516906 women (194079 aged 40–49, 171902 aged 50–59, 103451 aged 60–69, 41296 aged 70–79, 6030 aged 80–89, and 148 aged 90–96) with a total of 9116783 person years of follow-up (1970–1989) and 149044 deaths from all causes. The group of married women aged 80 or more were a strongly selected group because their husbands should be still alive. There were no married couples, aged 97 or more alive in 1970.

The statistical analyses were performed using SAS and GLIM statistical packages. Relative risks were computed in a generalised linear model based on Poisson distribution (Breslow and Day 1980) using the statistical package GLIM. Included in the analyses, as indicator variables, were age (six groups), education (two groups), number of children (five groups), age at first birth (three groups), and age at last birth (3 groups). The effect of any variable was judged by comparing the fit of models with and without the variable: the models included both main factors and interaction terms. The difference in fit of two models was tested by Chi-squared distributed statistics given as the difference between the deviance for the two models with k-1 degrees of freedom, where k was the number of levels of the factor.

Results

Tables 1 and 2 give a summary of the marital status in 1970 and total mortality rates (follow-up 1970–1989) for all women aged 20–99 (born 1871–1950) who participated in the 1970 Norwegian census. The proportion of never married women decreased from nearly 22 % in the age group 90– 99 to 7 % in women aged 30–39. In all age groups (except in women aged 90–99), the mortality rate was lowest in married women (Table 2).

Table 1. Marital status of women aged 20–99 in the 1970 Norwegian Census (N = 1338716)

Age group	Marital status				
	Married (%)	Widow (%)	Divorced/separated (%)	Not married (%)	Total
20–29	65.6	0.2	2.0	32.3	275261
30–39	88.8	0.9	3.1	7.1	197608
40–49	85.7	3.2	3.5	7.7	233463
50–59	76.4	9.3	3.8	10.6	242085
60–69	57.8	22.4	3.3	16.5	202927
70–79	34.9	41.9	2.9	20.3	135390
80–89	15.0	61.2	2.1	21.8	46743
90–99	3.7	72.9	1.7	21.8	5239

Table 2. Mortality rates per 100 person-years according to marital status of women aged 20–99 in the 1970 Norwegian census

Age group (years)	Marital status			
(years)	Married	Widow	Divorced/separated	Not married
20–29	0.0685	[a]	0.1462	0.0819
30–39	0.1756	0.2510	0.3220	0.3056
40–49	0.4543	0.5920	0.7311	0.7418
50–59	1.155	1.486	1.6234	1.490
60–69	3.239	3.765	3.9495	3.730
70–79	7.747	8.535	8.604	8.274
80–89	15.06	16.28	16.36	16.13
90–99	27.27	28.36	21.64	27.26

[a] only nine cases

The further analyses are restricted to married women (husband alive) who married before the age of 40 and with information about parity (Table 3). This represented 15 % of the age group 80–89 years and 4 % of the age group 90–96 years.

Higher education was set at eight years or more in the 1970 census. The proportion of women with eight years or more at school increased with decreasing

Table 3. Characteristics of married women aged 40–96 in the 1970 Norwegian census

	Age group (year)					
	40–49 (%)	50–59 (%)	60–69 (%)	70–79 (%)	80–89 (%)	90–96 (%)
Education						
7 years	51.1	61.4	66.2	73.9	80.5	85.8
8+ years	48.7	38.4	33.4	25.4	18.6	14.2
Parity (children)						
0	8.1	9.6	12.0	11.9	10.3	13.5
1	15.7	18.5	20.6	15.5	11.5	9.5
2	31.9	30.0	26.5	21.4	15.8	13.5
3	23.5	20.7	17.9	16.9	16.0	13.5
4–5	17.3	16.5	15.9	20.3	23.6	21.6
6+	3.6	4.8	7.0	14.1	22.8	28.4
Age at first birth						
< 24	42.0	30.6	32.2	38.9	28.4	16.7
25–34	52.3	59.8	52.9	51.4	60.5	71.4
35+	5.7	9.6	14.9	9.7	11.2	11.9
Age at last birth						
< 24	6.5	4.1	6.2	5.2	2.0	2.4
25–34	55.8	47.5	36.9	44.1	30.7	18.3
35+	37.7	48.5	56.9	50.7	67.3	79.4

age. Only 15 % of the women aged 90 or more in 1970 had higher education, compared with nearly half the women aged 40–49.

The fertility pattern differed according to age in this cohort (Table 3). More than 13 % of the women in the age group 90–96 were nullipara compared with 8 % in the age group 40–49. The number of women with six or more children dropped from 28 % to nearly 4 %. The portion of women who gave birth to their first child before the age of 25 increased from slightly more than 15 % in the oldest age group to more than 40 % in the youngest age group. Age at first and last birth revealed that women aged 60–69 years (born in 1901–1910) delayed their childbearing period to a higher age compared to both the older and younger age groups. Slightly more than 15 % of the women aged 90–96 gave birth before the age of 25, but nearly 80 % continued to give birth until after the age of 35. Nearly 15 % of the women in the age group 60–69 gave birth to their first child after the age of 35, but in both the older and the younger women this proportion was lower. In the age group 70–79 years, nearly 40 % had their first child before the age of 25, dropping to about 30 % in women aged 50–69 and rising to about 40 % in the youngest age group. The same trend was seen for age at last birth, where

Table 4. Age-specific total mortality per 100 years of observation, relative risk (RR) with 95 % confidence interval (95 % CI). Married women aged 40–96 in the 1970 Norwegian census with a follow-up in 1970–1989

| | Married | |
Age group (years)	Nulliparous	Parous
40–49		
Rate	0.6588	0.4304
RR	1.53	1.00 (reference)
95 % CI	1.46–1.60	
50–59 years		
Rate	1.1440	1.103
RR	1.26	1.00 (reference)
95 % CI	1.26–1.34	
60–69 years		
Rate	3.473	3.173
RR	1.09	1.00 (reference)
95 % CI	1.06–1.12	
70–79 years		
Rate	7.888	7.695
RR	1.02	1.00 (reference)
95 % CI	0.99–1.06	
80–89		
Rate	16.62	14.82
RR	1.10	1.00 (reference)
95 % CI	1.02–1.20	
90–96		
Rate	32.26	26.67
RR	1.16	1.00 (reference)
95 % CI	0.72–1.86	

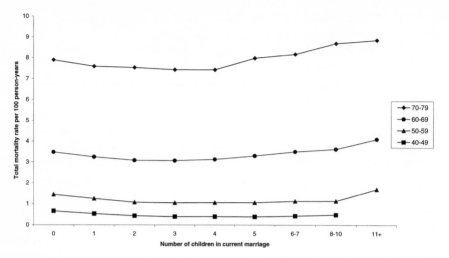

Fig. 1. Mortality per 100 years of observation by age group and parity. Married women aged 40–79 in the 1970 Norwegian census, with follow-up from 1970–1989. Covering 9 076 273 person-years with 142 905 deaths from all causes. N = 510 728

more than 55 % of the women aged 60–69 (born in 1900–1909) had their last child after the age of 34 compared with nearly 40 % among the youngest women.

Married nulliparous women had higher mortality rates than married parous women in all age groups (Table 4). Nulliparous women aged 40–49 years had a relative risk (RR) of 1.53 ([95 % confidence interval 1.46–1.60]). The effect of nulliparity decreased with increasing age group from 40–79, but rose again in women aged 80–96.

Age specific total mortality according to number of children gave a slightly u-shaped curve (Fig. 1). Nulliparous women and women with six or more children had higher mortality rates than women with two to five children. The same u-shaped curves were found after stratification on education (Fig. 2). Women with low education had higher mortality rates than women with higher education in all age groups and for all numbers of children.

Figure 3 shows a stratified analysis of parous women, including parity and age at first and last birth. Within each 10 year age group at the start of follow-up, the mortality rate is given for two strata according to age at first and last birth: those with all their births before the age of 25 years, and those with all their births after the age of 35 years. The analysis was restricted to women with one to five children. We found a strong interaction with age. The relative risk was highest in women with only early births, especially in the middle age groups, 50–59 and 60–69 years. Among the oldest we saw almost no differences in mortality rates with different childbearing patterns.

A multivariate Poisson regression analysis (Table 5) was used for calculation of RR with 95 % CI for death from all causes according to different fertility patterns and education. Higher education gave a risk reduction compared with

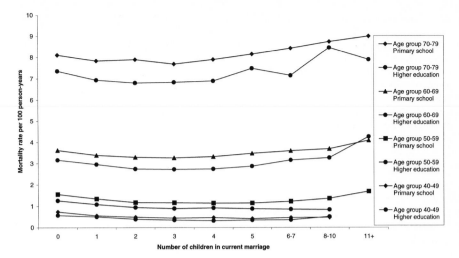

Fig. 2. Mortality per 100 years of observation by age group and parity. Married women aged 40–79 in the 1970 Norwegian census, with follow-up from 1970–1989. Covering 9 076 273 person-years with 142 905 deaths from all causes. N = 510 728

lower education of RR = 0.84, 95 % CI (0.83–0.85). Number of children gave a slightly u-formed curve in women with one to six children, where three children gave the lowest risk: RR = 0.92, 95 % CI (0.90–0.94). No consistent trend was found for age at first birth and mortality. For age at last birth, the relative risk decreased with increasing age: RR = 0.89, 95 %CI (0.87–0.92) in women aged 35 or more at last birth compared with women aged less than 24 at their last birth.

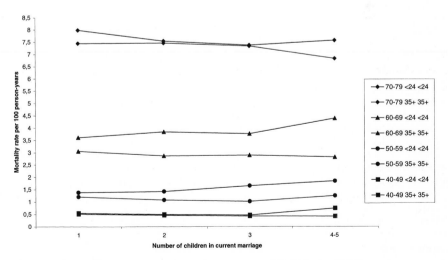

Fig. 3. Total mortality per 100 person-years in women agend 40–79 in the 1970 Norwegian census age at first and last birth

Table 5. Relative risk (RR) with 95 % confidence interval (95 % CI) for death from all causes according to fertility patterns and education in parous women 40–96 years. Poisson regression analysis with only singles terms. All variables are mutually adjusted for each other and for age

	RR	95 % CI
Education (years at school)		
7	1.0 (reference)	
8+	0.84	0.83–0.85
Parity (no. of children)		
1	1.0 (reference)	
2	0.94	0.92–0.95
3	0.92	0.90–0.94
4–5	0.95	0.93–0.97
6+	1.03	1.01–1.06
Age at first birth		
< 24	1.0 (reference)	
25–34	0.96	0.94–0.97
35+	0.98	0.96–1.01
Age at last birth		
< 24	1.0 (reference)	
25–34	0.95	0.92–0.97
35+	0.89	0.87–0.92

Table 6. Goodness-of-fit statistics (deviances) for different models fitted to total mortality data for Norwegian married women aged 40–79 at the 1970 census. Follow-up through 1970–1989

Factors in model	Deviance	d.f [a]	Change in deviance	d.f [a]
Total	130 144	289		
Single term added				
+ age	2 122.9	284	−128 021.1	5
+ education	1 134.1	283	−988.8	1
+ parity	925.0	279	−209.1	4
+ age at first birth	782.4	277	−142.6	2
+ age at last birth	709.2	275	−73.2	2
The terms of interaction added				
+ age * parity	524.0	255	−185.2	20
+ age * education	475.8	250	−48.2	5
+ age * age at first birth	423.3	240	−52.5	10
+ age * age at last birth	366.0	230	−57.3	10
+ parity * education	356.0	226	−10.0	4
+ parity * age at first birth	338.9	218	−17.1	8
+ parity * age at last birth	328.5	212	−10.4	6
+ age at first birth * age at last birth	324.5	210	−4.1	2
+ education * age at first birth	320.4	208	−4.1	2
+ education * age at last birth	319.4	206	−1.0	2

[a] Degrees of freedom

The fit of the model used for the estimation of relative risks is given in Table 6. Additional analyses of interactions confirmed the importance of the historical changes in childbearing pattern since all terms of interaction with age were highly significant (Table 6.).

Discussion

In this study of total mortality in a cohort of married Norwegian women, longevity is associated with a childbearing pattern of two to five children, born late in the fertile period. "Low age" at first birth does not favour a long life, but "high age" at last birth is significantly related to lower mortality.

Strength of Design

The 1970 Norwegian census was complete with almost no missing data (census officials visited every household to deliver and subsequently collect the pre-printed questionnaire); people who refused to co-operate were fined. The follow-up is complete and based on the unique identification number and national registers. The Norwegian population in 1970 was relatively ethnically homogeneous and stable with little immigration and a low rate of divorce.

The 1970 Norwegian census collected information about parity and age at first and last birth in married women (husband alive). This information about age in relation to parity permits us to analyse mortality not only in relation to parous/not parous women, but also in relation to number of children and age at first and last births. Age of children was not included in the census before 1970.

The main analyses were restricted to currently married women (husband alive), aged 40–96 years in 1970 (born 1874–1930), and who married before the age of 40 years. These women had mostly passed their childbearing period. The average additional number of children born to these women after the age of 40 years was less than 0.1 per woman. This gives a small, almost negligible, misclassification bias. Altering the age at marriage to < 35 years did not have a significant effect on the results (Lund 1990). Pregnancy-related deaths were negligible.

Weakness of Design

Lack of information about parity of the whole female cohort, independently of current civil status, left us unable to make a complete analysis, stratified on civil status, of longevity according to different patterns of childbearing. But it is possible that a cohort consisting of only married women is strengthened by greater homogeneity.

Selection based on marriage might lead to problems. Mortality rates were higher in unmarried than in married women. If childbearing had different effects depending on whether the mother was married or not, this would give biased estimates. The question about the number of children refers to children with the current husband; i.e., the women might have had children in a previous marriage or outside of marriage. Without the relevant information, we cannot control for these variables.

Before 1970, few couples in Norway became divorced; the rate was estimated to be about 20 per 10 000 marriages per year (Dyrvik 1976), and only about 5 % of all children in the period 1900–1970 were born to unmarried women (Statistics Norway 1985). Some of these women may have married later and reported a number of children in the current marriage that was lower than their actual fertility. This possibly might introduce some misclassification, but the effect is negligible. Analyses restricted to women who married before the age of 25 years did not change the conclusions (data not shown).

Because women's life expectancy was higher than men's, the proportion of married women decreased in the higher age groups, which meant that women in the higher age groups in our material were selected depending on whether or not they had married a healthy man. We do not know whether this selection bias affects the results.

Confounding Factors

Unfortunately, information on other important life style risks like smoking, diet, etc., which are important risk factors for death, was not collected in the 1970 Norwegian census. We are not able to correct for the confounding these risks might cause. The effect of parity on total mortality could be a social class effect; traditionally women with lower education have different fertility patterns than women with higher education. We have adjusted for education. Parity is still a protecting factor after adjusting for education, but we do not know whether residual confounding remains.

Other Studies

Since Williams' theory, called the pleiotropy theory was published in 1957 (Williams 1957), many evolutionary theories on ageing have been published. Most of the research on patterns of reproduction in relation to longevity has been done on animals like fruitflies. Only a few published papers are based on studies of human beings.

In 1985 Beral published a paper about the long-term effects of childbearing on health. She found that parous and nulliparous women had different panoramas of diseases. In this material parous women had a higher overall mortality than nulliparous women did, they lacked information about number of children and age at first or last birth.

Three years later Green et al. (1988) found that nulliparous women had higher mortality than parous women. However, they had no information about the women's age at childbirth.

Westendorp and Kirkwood (1998) found that number of progeny was negatively correlated with female longevity and age at first birth was positively correlated with longevity among women in the British aristocracy who lived to 60 years and more.

Pearls et al. (1997) found that centenarians were four times more likely to have had children after the age of 40 than women, who survived only to the age of 73, but their material consisted of very few old people, i.e. there was a lack of statistical power.

Le Bourg et al (1993) were not able to verify the prediction of a trade-off between early fecundity and longevity derived from Williams (1957) evolutionary theory of senescence in the analyses of the reproductive life of French-Canadian women in the 17–18th centuries.

Interpretation of our Findings

In this analysis with an extended follow-up period, we found that total mortality is associated with the pattern of childbearing. Total mortality is the sum of different specific mortality rates. In this presentation, we have not looked at different causes of death. The positive effect of postponed childbearing on mortality might be explained in many different ways. It should be noted that even though the decreased risks are small they have an important impact on longevity since we are dealing with total mortality over most of the life span.

The disposal soma theory on the evolution of ageing states that longevity requires investment in somatic maintenance, which reduces the resources available for reproduction. This theory suggests that there might be a trade-off between reproductive success and longevity, because resources invested in longevity assurance may be at the expense of reproduction (Kirkwood 1977; Kirkwood et al. 1991). Thus, women with low fertility will live longer than women with high fertility. If reproduction is at the cost of longevity, the result will be the same whether her fertility is high or low if her fecundity is low, i.e., she has few pregnancies. Low fecundity might be a result of low fertility, but can also be a result of cultural and non-biological explanations.

Late childbearing might indicate biologically slow ageing due to certain genes that might be associated with longevity (Perls et al. 1997). Alternatively, the positive effect of a late last birth could be due to an oestrogen peak late in life, which could protect for years to come against cardiovascular diseases and other causes of death, i.e., a hormonal explanation. This possibility could have an important impact on total mortality.

Further, women with a late last childbearing could be a selected group of women in relation to other aspects of life. If late childbearing is linked to less smoking, better social conditions, etc. then we have just observed a confounder.

There is a broad variety of evolutionary theories on ageing, and many scientists favour evolutionary explanations without considering alternative non-evolutionary theories fitting the given data just as well. An exception to this trend is Eric Le Bourg (1998).

Future Analyses

It is possible to make analyses of different specific mortality causes, and we think that these analyses should be based on a possible effect of a genetic hypothesis on each cause of death. It is also possible to carry out similar analyses on the husbands in the 1970 Norwegian cohort, which should enable us to improve our scrutiny of the effect of social class and help us to make a distinction between biology and life style factors (Kravdal 1995).

The findings from this study might have interesting implications for the young generation of Norwegian women, who spend an increasing number of years on education and give birth to one to three children late in their fertile period, after they have finished school. In 1998, the mean age at first birth was 28.8 years in married women (Statistics Norway 1999), which is very high in historical terms. The same situation applies in many European countries and could be an explanation for the increasing life expectancy among women.

We conclude that women with few children born late in the fertile period have the lowest mortality rate for the rest of their lives.

References

Beral V (1985) Long term effects of childbearing on health. J Epidemiol Community Health 39(4):343–346

Breslow NE and Day NE, (1980) Statistical methods in cancer research. Lyon: International Agency for Research on Cancer

Brunborg H (1988) Cohort and period fertility in Norway 1845–1985. 88/4

Dyrvik S (1976) Marriages and number of children-analyses of fertility trends in Norway 1920–1970. Central Bureau of Statistics. Article 89

Green A, Beral V, Moser K (1988) Mortality in women in relation to their childbearing history. Brit Med J 297(6645):391–395

Kirkwood TB (1977) Evolution of ageing. Nature 270(5635):301–304

Kirkwood TB, Rose MR (1991) Evolution of senescence: late survival sacrificed for reproduction. Philos Trans Roy Soc Lond B Biol Sci 332(1262):15–24

Kravdal O (1995) Is the relationship between childbearing and cancer incidence due to biology or life-style? Examples of the importance of using data on men. Int J Epidemiol 24(3):477–484

Le-Bourg E (1998) Evolutionary theories of aging: handle with care. Gerontology 44:345–348

Le-Bourg E, Thon B, Legare J, Desjardins B, Charbonneau H (1993) Reproductive life of French-Canadians in the 17–18th centuries: a search for a trade-off between early fecundity and longevity. Exp Gerontol 28(3):217–232

Lund E, Arnesen E, Borgan JK, (1990) Pattern of childbearing and mortality in married women – a national prospective study from Norway. J. Epidemiol. Community. Health 44 (3) 237–240

Perls TT, Alpert L, Fretts RC (1997) Middle-aged mothers live longer. Nature 389:133

Promislow DEL (1998) Longevity and the barren aristocrat. Nature 396:719–720

Statistics Norway (1985) Statistical yearbook 1985

Statistics Norway (1999) Aktuelle befolkningstall 8/99

Vassenden K (1987) Folke og boligtellingene 1960, 1970 og 1980 (The census 1960, 1970 and 1980). Central Bureau of Statistics. Repport 87/2

Westendorp RGJ, Kirkwood TBL (1998) Human longevity at the cost of reproductive success. Nature 396:743–746

Williams GC (1957) Pleiotrophy; natural selection and the evolution of science. Evolution 11:398–411

Sex-Differences in the Evolution of Life Expectancy and Health in Older Age

D. J. H. Deeg

Abstract

Since the middle of the 19th century, there have been considerable gains in life expectancy at all ages, especially during the first two decades of the 20th century. Throughout this period, women have had greater survival chances than males. Nevertheless, there are some notable sex differences in survival gains. Male infant survival increased faster than female infant survival, indicating narrowing sex differentials. The opposite is observed for survival to older ages. For instance, female survival to ages 50 and 65 increased faster than male survival to these ages, indicating a widening sex differential. This finding raises a question: how do these differences in cohort survival history affect health and mortality at ages above 65 years?

The role of cohort survival history was examined as an explanatory factor for sex differences in three-year survival in older persons in two surveys on health and aging, the Dutch Longitudinal Study among the Elderly (DLSE, baseline 1955–1957) and the Longitudinal Aging Study Amsterdam (LASA, baseline 1992–93). Both surveys are based on representative samples across the Netherlands, stratified by age and sex, with over 2000 persons in the common age group of 65–84 years. Cohort survival history was expressed as the percentage surviving up to ages 1, 15, 40, 50, and 65 based on cohort survival tables of the birth cohorts included in the study.

Both in 1955–57 and in 1992–93, when controlling for number of chronic diseases, functional limitations, and self-rated health, multiple logistic regression models showed that survival was significantly associated with sex, indicating that females had better survival than males. Inclusion of cohort survival history in the model raised these Risk Ratios to values closer to 1. Inclusion of survival to age 1 in DLSE resulted in a reversal of the sex differential. In LASA, inclusion of survival to age 1 increased the Risk Ratio significantly, but did not bring about a reversal of the risk. Inclusion of survival to age 50 in both surveys resulted in sex being no longer significantly associated with survival.

The consistent findings in both surveys suggest that the more favorable cohort survival history of females explains part of the female over male advantage in survival in later life, given the same level of health. This is true even for the infant mortality experience of the cohort. The better survival of females at all ages appears to perpetuate itself in older age.

Robine et al. (Eds.)
Sex and Longevity: Sexuality, Gender,
Reproduction, Parenthood
© Springer-Verlag Berlin Heidelberg 2000

Introduction

Over the past century, life expectancy of western populations has increased tremendously. Many more people are reaching old age nowadays than in the late nineteenth century. The question is whether health in old age has kept up with the extension of the average life span.

It seems a reasonable proposition that the proportion of older persons in poor health at one point in time is determined by past mortality rates in the surviving cohort (Crimmins et al. 1997). However, no estimates exist on the extent to which past cohort survival history determines current health status, relative to other determinants of health status. One major determinant of health status in older age is sex. A well-known paradox is associated with sex: within age groups, health status is almost invariably better for older men than for older women (e.g., Verbrugge 1985; Baltes et al. 1998), whereas older women have better chances of survival than men (Manton 1988; Arber and Ginn 1991). This chapter addresses the question: to what extent can sex differences in health status and survival chances of older persons be explained in terms of the past survival experience of their cohorts?

Following a review of the development of life expectancy and cohort survival since the second half of the nineteenth century, the development of health status of older persons is discussed based on two surveys conducted 37 years apart, in 1955–57 and in 1992–93. Cohort survival and health status are then combined in an analysis of prospective survival of both cohorts surveyed.

Life Expectancy 1860–1990

The most common way to calculate life expectancy is based on age-specific mortality rates observed in one calendar year. According to this measure, life expectancy at birth for men in the Netherlands more than doubled from 35 years in 1860 to 74 years in 1990. In women, the increase was from 37 years to 81 years. The increase was not linear, but showed several so-called turning points, where the rate of increase changed significantly (Van Poppel et al. 1996). One such turning point was in 1859, just around the time when mortality statistics in the Netherlands became sufficiently reliable. In 1859, the rate of increase of life expectancy changed from negative to positive. During the period until the second turning point in 1926, there was one notable downward peak in the development of life expectancy, namely in 1918 due to the Spanish influenza. In 1926 the rate of increase in life expectancy slowed down. This still positive rate of increase stayed the same until 1958, with the exception of the last years of World War II, when a large downward peak was observed, especially in men. From the next turning point, 1958, the development of life expectancy differed for men and women. For women, the increase in life expectancy continued, but again at a slower pace. For men, from 1958–1970 the rate of increase was negative, after which period a rapid increase could be observed (Van Poppel et al. 1996).

The male-female difference in life expectancy also showed several turning points. Until 1898, male excess mortality increased from two to three years. After the turning point year 1898, the male-female difference decreased again until the turning point year 1927, when it was just over one year. From 1927, the male excess mortality rapidly became larger until it was as much as 6.7 years in 1975. The main causes of death that affected men much more than women in this period were cardiovascular diseases and lung cancer (Mackenbach 1993). The most recent turning point was in 1975, which marked the beginning of a period of slow decrease of the male-female gap in life expectancy (Van Poppel et al. 1996).

The measures of life expectancy that are based on age-specific mortality rates in one calendar year are basically artificial. When a newborn child grows older, at each specific age he will be exposed to the mortality rates for that age in the year that he reaches that age. Thus, his true life expectancy is based on all mortality rates that apply to his age during the years that he lives through. This is the basis for calculating cohort life-expectancy. The way of calculating implies that cohort-based life expectancy can only be known when a cohort has become almost or totally extinct. At present, this is possible for the cohorts born in the nineteenth century. As is to be expected because of the general decrease in mortality rates from 1859, the cohort-based life expectancy exceeded the period-based life expectancy by several years. For men, the difference was about three years. For women, the difference increased from about three years in 1860 to almost seven years in 1900 (Van Poppel et al. 1996). Clearly, the cohort-based life expectancies show the widening gap between male and female life expectancies even for cohorts born in the late nineteenth century, who reached their fifties and sixties during the height of the male excess mortality for cardiovascular diseases and lung cancer.

Measures of Cohort Survival History

To study the relation between the evolution of life expectancy and health in older age, measures of cohort survival history were derived from Dutch national cohort life tables for men and women born in each of the birth years 1862–1937, thus covering the years in which the mortality statistics became reliable through the year in which the youngest survey participant was born. The cohort life tables were provided by the Netherlands Interdisciplinary Demographical Institute (Tabeau et al. 1994). 1990 was the most recent year for which cohort life table data were available. Cohort survival history can be expressed by a series of measures indicated by the percentage of survivors until a fixed age. Since survival data for ages 53 and older are not available for all cohorts included in the study (born in 1937 or earlier), percentages of survivors to ages 1, 15, 40, and 50 are used as indicators of cohort survival history. Each measure of survival was introduced in the respective data sets as a characteristic of the participants by assigning to each individual subject the value of the cohort survival measure for his/her year of birth and sex.

Two Health Surveys

Data from two health surveys were used to determine to what extent sex differences in health status and survival chances of older persons can be explained in terms of the past survival experience of their cohorts. The oldest survey is the baseline cycle of the Dutch Longitudinal Study of health among the Elderly (DSLE), which dates back to 1955–57, just before the turning point year after which the rates of increase in period-based life expectancy for men and women started to diverge. The most recent survey is the baseline cycle of the Longitudinal Aging Study Amsterdam (LASA), which took place in 1992–93. Both studies are nationwide with representative samples of over two 2000 persons aged 65–84 years, either living in the community or in residential homes for the elderly. Both studies include data on health in terms of chronic diseases, functional limitations, self-rated health, and mortality.

Study Samples

The main characteristics of the two survey samples are presented in Table 1. Baseline data and response rates are described elsewhere in detail (Van Zonneveld 1961; Deeg and Westendorp-de Serière 1994). Our study focuses on the overlapping age ranges of 65–84 years at baseline with known vital status at the last probing date (DLSE: N = 2370; LASA: N = 2104). Both samples are age and sex stratified so that each five-year age group contains approximately equal numbers of men and women. The DLSE sample is taken from 374 general practices and includes older persons living in the community as well as in residential homes for the aged. The LASA sample is taken from 11 municipal registries and includes older persons living in the community as well as institutionalized older persons. To denote the historic time of the DLSE baseline, the year of 1956 is used, being the middle year of the baseline examination. To denote the historic time of the LASA baseline, the year 1993 is used, being the year in which two-thirds of the participants were examined.

Table 1. Main characteristics of two longitudinal studies on aging in the Netherlands

Dutch Longitudinal Study among the Elderly (DLSE)	
1955–1957	3149 persons examined, ages 65–99 years, by 374 general practitioners, age and sex stratified sample, nationwide, on physical and psycho-social health
1960–1962	First of six follow-up cycles
1983	Termination of study; ascertainment of vital status and date of death, 1 % still alive
Longitudinal Aging Study Amsterdam (LASA)	
1992–1993	3107 persons examined, ages 55–84 years, by 43 trained lay interviewers, age and sex stratified sample, 11 geographically representative communities, on physical, cognitive, emotional, and social functioning
1995–1996	First follow-up cycle; ascertainment of vital status and date of death
1998–1999	Second follow-up cycle; ascertainment of vital status and date of death

Measures

For comparative purposes, variables were selected that have similar content and wording in each study. Table 2 lists the variables selected. "*Climbing stairs*" was the only common variable indicating functional limitations. Response categories were "able without help" and "not able without help". This operational definition of functional limitations by one item only is rather limited. However, in a pilot study including nine functional limitation items, climbing stairs proved to have the greatest item-rest correlation, thus suggesting that this item out of all single items reflects functional limitations best (Smits et al. 1997). Both studies included a question on *self-rated health*. In DLSE, the response categories were "good", "fair", "poor"; in LASA, "excellent", "good", "fair", "sometimes good, sometimes poor", and "poor" (NCBS 1992). In both cases, this item was dichotomized between "good" and "fair", resulting in two categories: "good" and "less-than-good". Thus, in DLSE on either side of the dichotomy, there is one good and one less-than-good category; in LASA, one additional category is used on either side of the dichotomy. Four *chronic disease* categories were common to both studies: respiratory diseases, heart diseases, diabetes, and arthritis. Answers were coded as "no" or "yes." In DLSE, no questions were asked about important diseases such as stroke and cancer. The validity of the ascertainment of chronic diseases in DLSE was warranted because it was the respondent's general practitioner who coded the answers in the questionnaire. In LASA, respondents' self-reports were compared to information obtained from their general practitioners, and proved to be adequate (Kriegsman et al. 1996). For the purpose of this study, the

Table 2. Wording of variables selected that are common to both studies: Dutch Longitudinal Study among the Elderly (1956–1961) and Longitudinal Aging Study Amsterdam (1993–1996)

Indicator	DLSE	LASA
Functional limitation	Can you climb stairs?	Can you climb 15 steps up and down without stopping?
Self-rated health	How is your health? (subjective health experience)	How in general is your health?
Respiratory diseases	Do you suffer from asthma bronchialis, bronchitis, persistent coughing, lung ailment, pleuritis, blood spitting, lung tuberculosis?	Do you have chronic non-specific lung disease, asthma, bronchitis, lung emphysema?
Heart diseases	Do you suffer from heart ailment, pain in the heart area, pressure on the breast, shortness of breath?	Do you have or have you had a heart disease?
Diabetes	Do you suffer from sugar disease?	Do you have diabetes?
Arthritis	Do you suffer from any form of "rheumatism"?	Do you have worn off joints or arthrosis of knees, hips, or hands, or do you have joint infection?

number of chronic disease categories was summed into a comorbidity index. In both cohorts, *vital status,* including date of death, were ascertained periodically through municipal registries. Three years after baseline, 23.1 % in DLSE and 17.4 % in LASA had died.

Statistical Methods

Statistical analysis proceeded according to four steps. First, the cohort survival history of males and females was examined both graphically and by comparing means and standard deviations across the periods 1872–1892 and 1907–1927, the birth years of the cohorts under study. Second, prevalences of indicators of poor health were compared for men and women across the two surveys. For reasons of simplicity, all prevalences were weighted according to the age distribution of the Dutch population in 1956. Health differences between 1956 and 1993 were tested using the chi-square statistic. Third, the predictive ability of health indicators for three-year mortality in each cohort was examined using multiple logistic regression models, including age and sex. For each independent variable, risk ratios (RRs) and 95 % confidence intervals (CIs) were calculated. Fourth, two measures of cohort survival history (percent surviving to age 1 and age 50) were introduced as additional predictor variables of three-year mortality in both cohorts, and their impact on the risk ratio of sex for mortality was examined.

Results

Cohort Survival History

As examples of the development of cohort survival history, Figure 1 shows cohort survival to age 1 and to age 50 for men and women. The percentages of the population surviving increased steadily in the period under study. From 1862 to 1937, the percentage surviving to year 1 increased from 80 % to 96 %, and the percentage surviving to year 50 increased even from 50 % to 90 %. Thus, a substantial portion of the improvement in survival was due to reduction of infant mortality, but more than half of the improvement was due to mortality reductions at ages beyond infancy. Notably, the gap between male and female survival closed for survival to age 1, but widened for survival to age 50.

Comparisons of means and standard deviations of cohort survival to ages 1, 15, 40, 50, and 65 for the periods 1872–1892 and 1907–1927, respectively, highlight the improvement in survival (Table 3). The largest increase is seen for survival to age 65: 16 % for males and 25 % for females. Generally, the standard deviations are larger for the recent period than for the early period, indicating that in cohorts born just after the turn of the century, the rate of increase in survival was greater than in those born just before the turn of the century. Also, female survival to older ages showed a larger standard deviation than male survival, in particular to age 65 (early cohort) and to ages 40 and older (recent cohort), indicating that female survival improved faster than male survival to these ages.

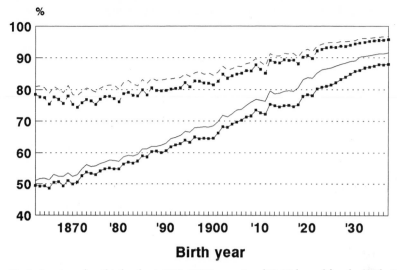

Fig. 1. Survivors from birth cohorts 1862–1937 to ages 1 and 50. Males and females in The Netherlands
Source: Netherlands Interdisciplinary Demographic Institute
----- To age 1, females
■-■ To age 1, males
—— To age 50, females
■■■ To age 50, males

Table 3. Measures of cohort survival, cohorts born 1872–1892 and 1907–1927, The Netherlands

| Cohort survival to age: | 1872–1892 | | | | 1907–1927 | | | |
| | Males surviving | | Females surviving | | Males surviving | | Females surviving | |
	Mean (%)	Standard deviation	Mean (%)	Standard deviation	Mean (%)	Standard deviation	Mean (%)	Standard deviation
1	78.1	1.4	81.4	1.3	89.6	2.4	91.8	2.2
15	67.0	2.0	70.2	1.9	84.4	3.4	86.9	3.4
40	59.8	2.3	62.6	2.1	79.3	3.5	83.5	4.0
50	56.7	2.6	59.0	2.5	76.6	3.4	81.6	4.0
65	45.7	2.4	48.9	3.0	62.2	3.0	73.7	3.6

Comparison of Health Status

A comparison of health indicators for the ages 65–84 years in the years 1956 and 1993, shows substantial differences, although not all in the same direction (Table 4). First, the prevalence of inability to climb stairs was greater in women than in men, and showed a relative decrease of 40 % in both men and women. This decrease is especially notable in view of the more strict wording of the question in LASA than in DLSE (Table 2). By contrast, the prevalence of less-than-

Table 4. Health status (%), standardized to the age distribution of the population in 1956

	DLSE 1956		LASA 1993	
	Males n = 1223	Females n = 1147	Males n = 1024	Females n = 1080
Stairs unable	12	28	7	17
Self-rated health < good	17	34	33	44
Heart diseases	15	20	26	16
Diabetes	4	7	8	9
Respiratary diseases	15	11	15	11
Arthritis	23	35	26	49
> = 2 diseases	11	16	16	19

Note: All prevalence differences between DLSE and LASA are significant (p < 0,05) except for respiratory diseases

good self-rated health showed a strong relative increase, as much as 87 % in men and 26 % in women. Despite the larger increase in men, in both periods women reported less-than-good health more often than men. The prevalence of heart diseases was greater in men than in women, and showed a relative increase of 77 % in men, whereas it showed a relative decrease of 18 % in women. The prevalence of diabetes was greater in women than in men in both periods, and rose in both sexes: the relative increase was as much as 105 % in men and 32 % in women. The prevalence of respiratory diseases was again greater in men than in women, and remained constant across the period. The prevalence of arthritis was substantially greater in women than in men, which difference became only larger due to a relative increase in prevalence of 13 % in men and 40 % in women. Finally, the prevalence of comorbidity (individuals having two or more diseases) was greater in women than in men in both periods, and showed a relative increase of 45 % in men and 19 % in women. In summary, in both periods, more health indicators showed poorer health for women as compared to men than the reverse.

Predictors of Three-Year Mortality

In both cohorts, three-year mortality was clearly lower for women than for men (Table 5a). Controlling for the other predictors, women's chances of dying in the next three years were only 66 % of men's in DLSE and only 38 % of men's in LASA (RR = 0.66 and 0.38, respectively). The sex difference in mortality was significantly greater in LASA (the RR of 0.38 in LASA lying outside the confidence interval for the RR of 0.66 in DLSE), corresponding to the larger increase in survival in women at ages younger than 65, noted above. Of course, mortality increased with age: by 9–10 % per year in both cohorts. Health indicators that predicted mortality in both cohorts were the number of chronic diseases and the number of functional limitations. Self-rated health was strongly predictive in DLSE, but showed no predictive ability for mortality in LASA.

Table 5a. Predictors of three-year mortality, 1956–1959 and 1993–1996: baseline health status

	DLSE 1956 OR (95 % CI)	LASA 1993 OR (95 % CI)
Sex (female vs male)	0.66 (0.53 – 0.82)	0.38 (0.29 – 0.50)
Age (years)	1.10 (1.07 – 1.12)	1.09 (1.06 – 1.12)
No. of chronic diseases	1.20 (1.04 – 1.37)	1.20 (1.07 – 1.35)
No. of functional limitations	1.57 (1.40 – 1.78)	1.36 (1.22 – 1.51)
Self-rated health	1.91 (1.50 – 2.43)	0.98 (0.74 – 1.31)

Table 5b. Predictors of three-year mortality, 1956–1959 and 1993–1996: cohort survival history

	DLSE 1956 OR (95 % CI)	LASA 1993 OR (95 % CI)
Cohort survival to age 1[a]	0.77 (0.71 – 0.83)	0.82 (0.78 – 0.87)
Cohort survival to age 50[b]	0.84 (0.80 – 0.88)	0.87 (0.83 – 0.90)

[a] Adjusted for sex, chronic disease, functional limitations, self-rated health

Table 5c. Predictors of three-year mortality, 1956–1959 and 1993–1996: sex and cohort survival history

	DLSE 1956 OR (95 % CI)	LASA 1993 OR (95 % CI)
Sex[a]	0.64 (0.51 – 0.79)	0.37 (0.12 – 0.62)
Sex[a] + cohort survival to age 1	1.66 (1.17 – 2.36)	0.58 (0.44 – 0.76)
Sex [a] + cohort survival to age 50	0.99 (0.77 – 1.26)	0.68 (0.51 – 0.91)

[a] Adjusted for chronic disease, functional limitations, self-rated health

In a logistic regression model including all health indicators and sex[1] (Table 5b), cohort survival history appeared to have a relative risk of mortality that was significantly less than 1 in both DLSE and LASA: 0.77 and 0.82 for survival to age 1, and 0.84 and 0.87 for survival to age 50, respectively. For example

---

[1] Age was no longer included in the model, because its correlation with the cohort survival measures was too high (over 0.90), and would lead to multicollinearity

a relative risk of 0.77 means that, for each percentage point of better survival history, cohort members had only 77 % of the mortality risk. Note, that the relative risk was significantly lower for survival to age 1 than for survival to age 50 (both in DLSE and LASA, the RR for survival to age 50 was outside the CI interval for the RR for survival to age 1).

Finally, the addition of cohort survival history to the model raised the relative risk of sex for mortality to values closer to 1, and in one case (survival to age 1 in DLSE) to values greater than 1. In one case (survival to age 50 in DLSE), the contribution of sex to mortality was no longer significant. In all cases, the RR of sex after inclusion of cohort survival history into the model differed significantly from the RR of sex before inclusion of cohort survival history into the model. This is a remarkable finding, indicating that the sex difference in mortality after age 65 can be attributed partly to the better cohort survival history of women before age 50.

Conclusions

With respect to cohort survival history, the analyses described in this chapter lead to the following conclusions:
1) Life expectancy as well as cohort survival improved in all phases of life.
2) Since 1862, cohort survival was more favorable in women than in men.
3) The sex differential in cohort survival to age 1 *decreased*.
4) The sex differential in cohort survival to ages above 50 *increased*.

Thus, generally, recent history has favored women more than men in terms of survival chances. However, whether this better survival has also brought better health to older women is doubtful. Examination of the sex differential in health status showed that comorbidity was greater in women in both periods, in particular due to diabetes and arthritis, and increased across time. Correspondingly, in both periods women more often were unable to climb stairs than men, although the prevalence of inability to climb stairs decreased across time. Women also reported less-than-good health more often than men in both periods, the prevalence of which *in*creased over time.

The poorer baseline health status of women aged 65–84 years in both periods studied did not prevent the sex differential in three-year survival from *in*creasing over time. Moreover, cohort survival history was positively associated with prospective three-year survival, and the more favorable cohort survival history of females as compared to males explained part of the female-over-male advantage in survival in later life, given the same level of health. This was true even for the infant mortality experience of the cohort. One might conclude that the better survival of females at all ages appears to perpetuate itself in older age, to the detriment of the health of older females.

The association found between cohort survival history and the sex differential in mortality in old age may be due to a confounding factor that affects both the cohort survival history and the sex differential in mortality. One candidate confounder might be the fertility of women, which decreased across the period studied. Further research is warranted to examine the relation between fertility, cohort survival history, and the sex differential in mortality (see Kirkwood, elsewhere in this volume).

A more straightforward explanation of the association between cohort survival history and the sex differential in mortality in old age may be based on the observed difference between the development of the male-female gap in survival to age 1 and to age 50. The convergence of the former gap may save frail males from infant mortality, only to die with greater probability in middle and old age, thus widening the latter gap. However, the extent of the convergence of the sex differential in survival to age 1 is too small to account for all of the sex differential in survival to older ages.

The findings of this study also suggest that, to further explain the sex differential in longevity, one has to look for mechanisms at work around birth, through adulthood, *and* in old age. Alternatively, there could be different but related mechanisms for each phase of life. Or again there may be mechanisms that produce "survival attributes" early in life, which attributes gain in importance as individuals age (Vaupel et al. 1998). Several possible explanations for the sex differential in longevity have been been put forward, from purely biological to purely social:

1) Differences in regulation of energy balance (Koistinen et al. 998), immune response related to sex hormones (Whitacre et al. 1999), heart rate dynamics (Ryan et al. 1994) – resulting in differences in disease etiology, susceptibility for risk factors, and disease incidence (Ory and Warner 1990)
2) Differences in reproductive strategy (Vinogradov 1998)
3) Differences in amount of stress
4) Differences in life style or health habits
5) Differences in timing and anticipation of life course events, in particular losses (Barer 1994)
6) Differences in coping with stressful life events (Henrard 1996)
7) Regular supervision by doctors, starting from menarche (Lagro-Jansen 1997; Verbrugge 1990)
8) Differences in social integration and social protection (Hessler et al. 1995).

Of these explanations, the behavioral and social ones clearly pertain only to later phases of the life course and not to infancy. Nor do they seem related to the biological explanations. Thus, these would not explain satisfactorily why cohort survival history to age 1 can account for the sex differential in survival after age 65. The first explanation does cover all phases of life, as do the second and third if they are understood in a purely biological sense. In conclusion, then, it is towards these most promising explanations that endeavors to understand the sex differential in longevity should be directed.

References

Arber S, Ginn J (1991) Gender, class, and health in later life. In: Arber S, Ginn J (eds) Gender and later life. A sociological analysis of resources and constraints. London, Sage Publications, 107–128

Baltes MM, Freund AM, Horgas AL (1998) Men and women in the Berlin Aging Study. In: Baltes PB, Mayer KU (eds) The Berlin aging study, Aging from 70 to 100. Cambridge, Cambridge University Press, 259

Barer BM (1994) Men and women aging differently. Int J Aging Human Dev 38:29–40

Crimmins EM, Saito Y, Reynolds S (1997) Further evidence on recent trends in the prevalence and incidence of disability among older Americans from two sources: the LSOA and the NHIS. J Geront Soc Sci 52B:S59–S71

Deeg DJH, Westendorp-de Serière M (eds) (1994) Autonomy and well-being in the aging population I: Report from the Longitudinal Aging Study Amsterdam 1992–1993. Amsterdam: VU University Press (ISBN 90-5383-336-6)

Henrard JC (1996) Cultural problems of aging especially regarding gender and intergenerational equity. Soc Sci Med 43:667–680

Hessler RM, Jia S, Madsen R, Pazaki H (1995) Gender, social networks and survival time – a 20-year study of the rural elderly. Arch Gerontol Geriat 21:291–306

Koistinen HA, Koivisto VA, Karonen S, Ronnemaa T, Tilvis RS (1998) Serum leptin and longevity. Aging: Clin Exp Res 10:449–454

Kriegsman DMW, Penninx BWJH, Van Eijk JTM, Boeke AJP, Deeg DJH (1996) Self-reports and general practitioner information on the presence of chronic diseases in community-dwelling elderly. A study on the accuracy of patients' self-reports and on determinants of inaccuracy. J Clin Epidemiol 49:1407–1417

Largro-Jansen T (1997) De tweeslachtigheid van het verechil [The ambiguity of the difference]. Nijmegen, The Netherlands:SUN

Mackenbach JP (1993) The epidemiologic transition in the Netherlands [De epidemiologische transitie in Nederland]. Nederlands Tijdschrift voor Geneeskunde 137:132–8

Manton KG (1988) A longitudinal study of functional change and mortality in the United States. J Gerontol 43 (Suppl 5):S153–S161

Netherlands Central Bureau of Statistics (NCBS) (1992) Netherlands Health Interview Survey 1981–1991. The Hague, The Netherlands: SDU Publishers/CBS Publications

Ory MG, Warner HR (1990) End notes: Closing the gender gap? Need for further research. In: Ory MG, Warner HR (eds). Gender, health, and longevity. Multidisciplinary perspectives. New York, Springer, 255–257

Ryan SM, Goldberger AL, Pincus S, Mietus J, Lipsitz LA (1994) Gender- and age-related differences in heart rate dynamics: Are women more complex than men? J Am Coll Cardiol 24:1200–1207

Smits CHM, Deeg DJH, Jonker C (1997) Cognitive and emotional predictors of disablement in older adults. J Aging Health 9:204–221

Tabeau E, Van Poppel F, Willekens F (1994) Mortality in The Netherlands 1850–1991. The data base. The Hague, Netherlands Interdisciplinary Demographic Institute

Van Poppel F, Tabeau E, Willekens F (1996) Trends and sex-differentials in Dutch mortality since 1850: Insights from a cohort- and period-perspective. GENUS LII:107–134

Van Zonneveld RJ (1961) The health of the aged. Assen, The Netherlands, Van Gorcum

Vaupel JW, Carey JR, Christensen K, Johnson TE, Yashin A, Holm NV, Iachine IA, Kannisto V, Khazaeli AA, Liedo P, Longo VD, Zeng Y, Manton KG, Curtsinger JW (1998) Biodemographic trajectories of longevity. Science 280:855–860

Verbrugge LM (1985) Gender and health: An update on hypotheses and evidence. J Health Soc Behav 26:156–182

Verbrugge LM (1990) Pathways of health and death. In: Apple RD (ed) Women, health, and medicine in America. A historical handbook. New York, Garland, 41–79

Vinogradov AE (1998) Male reproductive strategy and decreased longevity. Acta Biotheor 46:157–160

Whitacre CC, Reingold SC, O'Looney PA (1999) Task force on gender, multiple sclerosis and autoimmunity. A gender gap in autoimmunity. Science 283:1277–1278

Subject Index